FINDING THE NEW YOU

FINDING THE NEW YOU

THINK, SEE, AND FEEL BEAUTIFUL

DENNIS SCHIMPF MD, MBA, FACS

ForbesBooks

Published by ForbesBooks, Charleston, South Carolina.
Member of Advantage Media Group.

ForbesBooks is a registered trademark, and the ForbesBooks colophon is a trademark of Forbes Media, LLC.

Printed in the United States of America.

10 9 8 7 6 5 4 3 2 1

ISBN: 978-1-950863-30-3
LCCN: 2021908153

Cover design by Carly Blake.
Layout design by Megan Elger.

This custom publication is intended to provide accurate information and the opinions of the author in regard to the subject matter covered. It is sold with the understanding that the publisher, Advantage|ForbesBooks, is not engaged in rendering legal, financial, or professional services of any kind. If legal advice or other expert assistance is required, the reader is advised to seek the services of a competent professional.

Advantage Media Group is proud to be a part of the Tree Neutral® program. Tree Neutral offsets the number of trees consumed in the production and printing of this book by taking proactive steps such as planting trees in direct proportion to the number of trees used to print books. To learn more about Tree Neutral, please visit **www.treeneutral.com**.

Since 1917, Forbes has remained steadfast in its mission to serve as the defining voice of entrepreneurial capitalism. ForbesBooks, launched in 2016 through a partnership with Advantage Media Group, furthers that aim by helping business and thought leaders bring their stories, passion, and knowledge to the forefront in custom books. Opinions expressed by ForbesBooks authors are their own. To be considered for publication, please visit **www.forbesbooks.com**.

Dedicated to my mother, Jean, and my father, Dennis.

My mother had a contagious smile and boundless generosity. She was taken from us far too soon, but I often think about her and the impact she had on me. My father is a strong, dedicated man whose hard work and discipline provided me opportunities for which I will forever be thankful. I strive to be more like him every day. Although neither of my parents pursued higher education, they are great examples of how some of life's most important lessons cannot always be learned in the classroom.

CONTENTS

ABOUT THE AUTHOR

Dennis Schimpf, MD, MBA, FACS, practiced plastic surgery as a full-time faculty member for five years at the Medical University of South Carolina (MUSC) before starting his own private practice, Sweetgrass Plastic Surgery, in 2013. While his initial focus of practice at MUSC was reconstruction following a mastectomy, abdominal wall reconstruction after hernia repair, and cleft lip/palate surgery, in private practice he focuses exclusively on cosmetic plastic surgery of the face and body.

Dennis is board certified by the American Board of Plastic Surgery and is a fellow of the American College of Surgeons (FACS), as well as a member of the American Society of Aesthetic Plastic Surgery (ASAPS) and the American Society of Plastic Surgery (ASPS). While at MUSC, he founded and directed the Advanced Breast Reconstruction Program at the NCI-designated Hollings Cancer Center. Dennis also has an MBA from the Darla Moore School of Business at the University of South Carolina with a concentration in international business.

Sweetgrass Plastic Surgery has multiple offices throughout Charleston, South Carolina, where Dennis and his team annually perform over two thousand cosmetic plastic surgery procedures of the face and body, including approximately one thousand procedures using general IV sedation in their office operating rooms.

A side passion for Dennis is Pedals 4 Peanuts, an organization he founded during Christmas 2013 to provide new bicycles and helmets for underprivileged kids in conjunction with local police departments after he saw the excitement in the eyes of his youngest daughter, nicknamed Peanut, when she got her first bike. The charity has given away over nearly twenty-five hundred new bikes and helmets since its inception.

Dennis is also the founder of Loopit, a revolutionary cloud-based patient engagement and review platform focused on improving the quality of the review process for businesses and patients within the health and wellness industry. Dennis and his wife, Lori, have seven children and live on Daniel Island in Charleston, South Carolina.

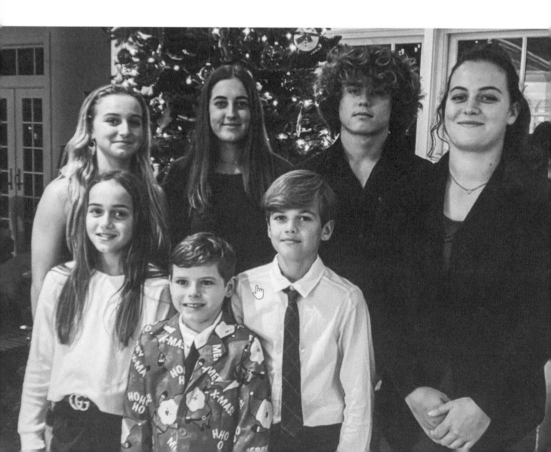

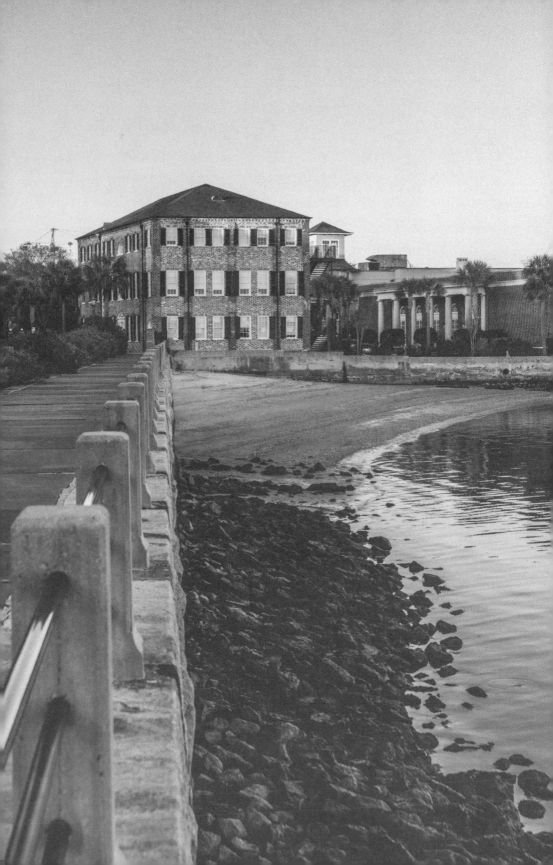

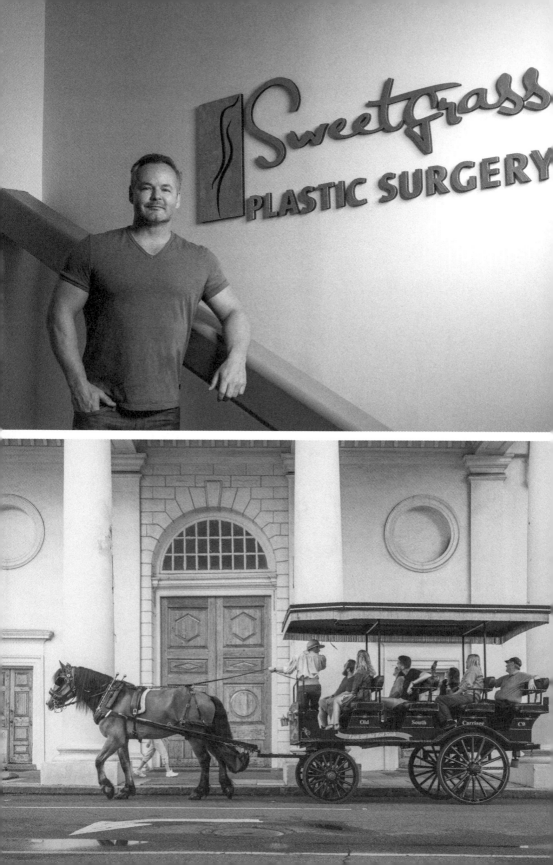

FOREWORD

Dennis has been my best friend for over three decades. We met when we both played Little League baseball together at thirteen years of age. We grew up in the same town and were both starting guards for our senior year in high school, when he scored a lot and I fouled a lot. Dennis was the best man at my wedding, and I was at his. We stood by each other's sides when my father and his mother died too young. He is the godfather to my daughter, Claire, and I am the godfather to one of his daughters, Emma. Dennis and I also had very similar childhoods, growing up in a family of four. Both of our fathers served in and survived Vietnam. None of our parents have a four-year degree, but they defined who we are today.

Dennis became a successful plastic surgeon, businessman, and philanthropist, and I became a partner at an intellectual property law firm after obtaining a bachelor's degree in mechanical engineering and a law degree. A doctor and a lawyer. Sounds more like the beginning of a joke, and we all know the lawyer is going to be part of the punch line. However, what Dennis and I have accomplished through the years since that first encounter on the baseball diamond is no laughing matter. We have both worked hard to get where we are today. We also both specialized within the broader legal and medical professions.

In this book, Dennis explores the meaning of the word *beauty* in the realm of his profession of plastic surgery. Beauty is notoriously subjective and comes in a variety of forms. Dennis reminds us that beauty is not only recognized through appearance, but that it's an inner quality all of us have. Initially, anyone picking up this book may think the focus is on the improvement of the outward physical appearance sculpted by a talented plastic surgeon. However, Dennis explores the inner feelings driving a person's desire to change his or her outward appearance. Based on his own professional experiences, Dennis points out that, although plastic surgery may change your outward appearance, it will not change your emotional state and who you are on the inside unless you are comfortable with your decision and the outcome.

According to the American Society of Plastic Surgeons (ASPS), the number of cosmetic procedures continues to grow year after year. Many of these procedures, especially the minimally invasive ones, are performed by a variety of providers. Unfortunately, not all of the providers have the expertise or rigorous training of a plastic surgeon. As an experienced intellectual property lawyer, I encounter the same problem when general practice lawyers try to advise clients on a specialty they are not familiar with. Would anyone really use a real estate attorney to litigate a patent? Unfortunately, some people do. In this regard, Dennis offers invaluable advice and guidance from his many years of accomplished medical experience and thousands of procedures to ensure you are making the right decisions about plastic surgery.

Dennis walks us through every step of the process, from selecting the right doctor and the right procedure to preoperative risks and postsurgical expectations. He delivers valuable insight through real-world concerns and patient anecdotes, which helps achieve an optimal surgical decision that prepares a patient for making the right decision for the right reasons. This book should be part of every potential patient's homework in selecting a plastic surgeon and procedure. It reminds us that plastic surgery is not only about making you look better on the outside but also about feeling better and more confident about the process and reasons for surgery in the first place.

Similar to choosing the right lawyer, selecting the right plastic surgeon and treatment option is critical to physical and emotional success. I strongly recommend this book to any person considering plastic surgery. It will open your mind in your quest for beauty, whether it be when you look in the mirror or how you feel about who you are on the inside. I can say without reservation that this book, and more specifically, the author, is someone I would listen to. I have cherished his advice for more than three decades now and consider his friendship a part of my own success.

Brett M. Hutton

Partner
Heslin Rothenberg Farley & Mesiti P.C.
5 Columbia Circle, Albany, New York

"WHETHER IT'S
THE BEST OF TIMES
OR THE WORST OF
TIMES, IT'S THE ONLY
TIME WE'VE GOT."

—ART BUCHWALD

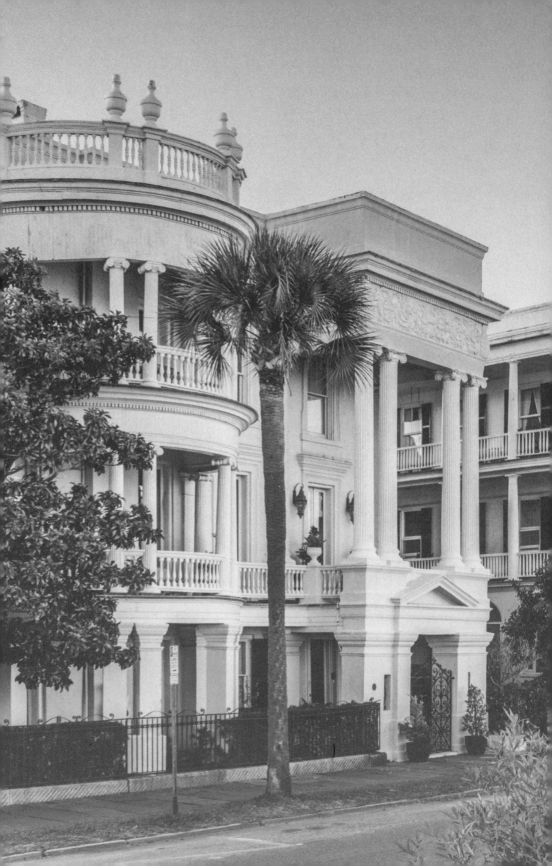

INTRODUCTION

*B*eauty is a word used to describe so many different things. It can describe a person, place, or object; it can describe an act toward a person or circumstance; it can describe a person's qualities. So while *beauty* often refers to physical attributes, it is also the emotional connection you have to a person, thing, or circumstance that makes you feel good.

The emotional or inner sense of beauty is not something you can see; it's something that touches you on the inside. It's like seeing a tiny baby. I'm a father many times over, but not one of my kids was what might be considered beautiful the moment they were born. When you get right down to it, newborns aren't that attractive; they can be a little goofy looking at best. But few adults can resist going a little gaga over any newborn. All that innocent newness can touch nearly any adult, making them well up with emotion. That doesn't happen because a baby is trying to look better for you; it happens because of how a baby makes you feel.

Take a moment to look at this drawing. What words would you use to describe it? Cute? Pretty? Simple?

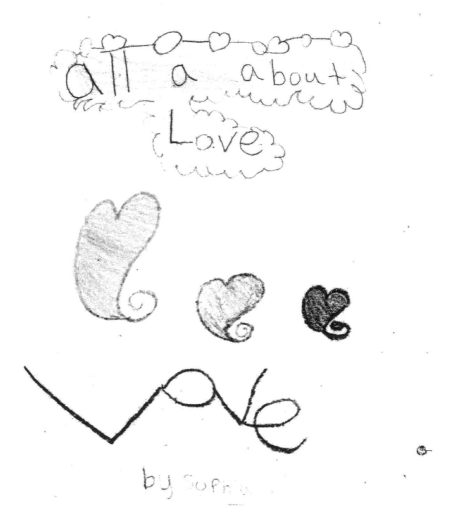

Most people would use words like those to describe it. No one would likely call it beautiful. However, what if I told you this was the last drawing a six-year-old girl did before she died of an illness? Is it beautiful now?

That inner feeling of beauty is the subject of a great many TED Talks, one of which I was listening to a few years ago while traveling from South Carolina, where I practice, to Florida. This particular talk was by a product designer, Richard Seymour, who explained that beauty is more than just what a person sees; it's about what a product makes a person feel. Something about his talk struck me, and I listened to it over and over again.

Part of what struck me was a simple, black-and-white line drawing of a flower and a butterfly created by a child. "Is it beautiful?" Seymour asks. Admittedly, there doesn't appear to be anything special about the drawing. Then Seymour explains its significance: initially, the drawing doesn't appear visually beautiful (see), and no one would use the term *beautiful* to describe it (think), but once viewers develop an emotional attachment to it, they find it to be truly beautiful (feel). That's what it means to *see*, *think*, and *feel* beauty.

While Seymour was talking about products from a design perspective, I realized there was some crossover to plastic surgery, my area of expertise. For example, the beauty of an automobile's appearance comes from the way its shape reflects light. Similarly, in the human face, wrinkles are basically created by shadows, so eliminating them is a matter of managing how they reflect light.

In addition, the face goes from an inverted, youthful triangular shape in youth to an upright triangular shape as a person ages and gravity causes tissue to descend. With age, the face becomes thin and elongated, as opposed to plump and round like the face of a young child. Ironically, these contour changes and vectors of the face are accentuated as they interact with light.

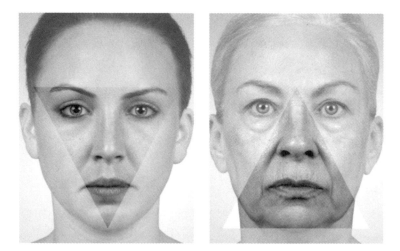

As I write this book, we're in the midst of the COVID-19 novel coronavirus pandemic and perhaps one of the most hostile political environments our country has ever known. You can see the look of despair in many of our patients on a daily basis. The pandemic and its catastrophic impacts on the economy, travel, education, and family life have been dramatic. Parents facing job uncertainty and being forced to fill in as teachers at home for their kids have taken a toll on everyone. In addition, not a day goes by in the office without a reference to the chaos of our political divide. These are strange times for most of us for sure. Interestingly, in a multitude of ways, this has made people more aware of how they appear and how they feel about themselves. I believe far more so now than before the pandemic, it's made them want to feel their best. It also seems to have brought to the surface a "live for the moment" mentality. People seem to want to do things that they wouldn't have done had this not happened, maybe because now they have a little more time to reflect, and they realize that life is short and things can change dramatically. Life has slowed down a little bit. They're not on the run as much, and they don't have dozens of things going on at once. In many ways they have more time to notice signs of aging. In fact, I often hear, "I had no idea I looked that old until I started having daily Zoom calls and I saw myself on camera." The digital age and technology are constantly reminding us of how we look, and as a result, it's become more important to people to look as good as they feel. In fact, the most common response I hear from a patient when I ask, "What is your overall goal in pursuing cosmetic plastic surgery?" is "To look as good as I feel." Also, many people have found themselves not having to show up at the office, so they are readily available to have a procedure done. For the first time, they don't have to worry about taking off from work, missing a trip or something they had scheduled, or coming into the office and having everyone ask about what they had done.

My purpose as a cosmetic plastic surgeon is to orchestrate physical change in a patient. However, I have found over time that there is a direct connection between what I do for a patient physically and the "inner beauty" the patient desires and ultimately achieves. The surgery alone does not change how you feel about yourself or the feelings others have when they see you. When a patient has self-doubt or insecurity as a result of a physical imperfection they see, surgery may have a profound impact on them. It is the combination of the physical change through the surgery and the patient's newfound self-confidence that makes their inner happiness project to those around them. That change is what ultimately makes a patient feel beautiful. I have seen that change quite often in young women who come in for breast augmentation after living their whole life with

> There is a direct connection between what I do for a patient physically and the "inner beauty" the patient desires and ultimately achieves.

smaller breasts. Once they have breasts that allow them to feel more confident in a swimsuit or other clothing, they tend to carry themselves differently. They're more confident, more vibrant. They are no longer timid and unsure of themselves in bathing suits or clothing. The surgery itself did not change *who* they were on the inside. But it can make you feel better and more beautiful. When you feel better and more beautiful, you project that happiness to others.

Plastic surgery has the potential to change virtually everything about a person on some level. Few things can single-handedly alter a person in such a way.

Over the years, some cases in particular have stuck with me as examples of how there are deeper facets to beauty.

One of those cases happened a few years after I had been in private practice. A twenty-five-year-old woman came into the office to see about getting a rhinoplasty (a nose job). After introducing myself and talking with her for a few minutes, she said, "I don't really like my nose."

As with every consult, I asked for more information: "Please tell me what you see that you don't like."

She couldn't really pinpoint what dissatisfied her. She just kept saying, "I don't know. I just don't like the way I look."

Finally, I told her, "Honestly, you have a nice-looking nose. There are some minor changes that could be made, but really, I do not think surgery is what you need." I often joke with patients in a scenario like this, saying, "I can only screw things up from here."

Without much of a pause, she then asked, "Well, what about my eyes?"

"Your eyes are beautiful," I told her truthfully. She really was a beautiful young woman.

At that point, her eyes began to well up, and she struggled to hold back the tears.

I paused while she tried to collect herself and then told her the truth: "I want to help you, but I have to really be able to see what it is about your features that you're upset with. Otherwise, I don't know what surgery I can offer that will help you."

At that, she burst into tears. After she calmed down and began collecting herself, she explained that her husband had told her that she wasn't as beautiful as he *needed* her to be. Think about that: *as beautiful as he needed her to be*. Imagine the impact on a twentysomething being told that by her husband. Young women, especially after having kids, are often so insecure about how they look and have so much self-doubt that a significant other's criticism has a brutal effect on their emotional state, on their psyche. They often don't feel beautiful in their own skin. I'm sure there are few things more painful that can be said to a woman in that situation.

I talked to her some more and tried to explain that there wasn't a surgery that was going to fix what was wrong with her situation. Even though I'm certain virtually any person seeing her would think she was beautiful, her husband did not see her that way, nor did she see it in herself. She ultimately admitted that she knew surgery wasn't the fix. What if surgery made her different but in a way that her husband found less attractive? There's a near guarantee that attempting to deliver results based on a third party's expectations will not be the answer. The young woman had come to me with the idea that she wanted to make the situation better, but surgery could have made the situation worse.

In the end, since her brother's wedding was coming up, she decided to have some topical skin-care treatments done, which made her feel better and more refreshed, with glowing skin and a renewed self-confidence.

That experience really underscores what plastic surgeons know: sometimes surgery is not the answer for what ails an individual.

For some people, beauty is only about physical attributes, and even that is a subjective judgment. For others, beauty is about who that person is within, and how that person makes others feel. Some see beauty, and others may think they see beauty, but ultimately, the goal is to feel it. That's what any person considering cosmetic plastic surgery must understand: Where is true beauty found? I believe that this simple yet critical principle is at the core of what ultimately makes a patient satisfied or unsatisfied with their choice to have surgery.

Helping people with their own definitions of beauty is something I strive to do every day as a plastic surgeon. I came to medicine comparatively late. I attended college on an athletic scholarship and planned to pursue a law degree after going through a master's degree program in student personnel administration. However, since I was

> That's what any person considering cosmetic plastic surgery must understand: Where is true beauty found?

lacking community service requirements needed to graduate, in the spring of my senior year, I volunteered in the emergency room of a local hospital. My college adviser had told me that the only way to get the hours I needed was to find someplace that was open twenty-four hours a day and put in a couple of days a week. Even though I was transporting patients, organizing supplies, cleaning floors, and doing whatever else needed to be done, I instantly enjoyed what I was doing there more than anything else I had done at school or in any job up to that point. That's when I decided that I wanted to go to medical school.

Since I had thus far taken very few science courses, the only way I could meet the prerequisites for medical school was to take an extra two years, concentrating on science and math classes. I made it through that grueling schedule with nearly straight As. Turned out I loved science and math and was pretty good at both subjects. That opened the door to medical school.

After graduating from medical school, I knew I wanted to train in surgery as my specialty, although I was unsure of a subspecialty. So as a resident, I did rotations in different kinds of surgery, ultimately deciding to focus on plastic surgery.

I spent five years in general surgery, after which I became board certified in general surgery. People always ask what made me choose surgery, the longest, most difficult, and most grueling of the training programs. I was drawn to the here-and-now aspect of it. Unlike family medicine, in which you prescribe a pill, wait a few weeks to see how it affects the patient, and then possibly change the medicine and wait again, I loved performing procedures, and when operating—especially when operating on a trauma patient—I could immediately see how my work was going to affect a patient. Operating inside a body, trying to cure patients and fix traumatic injuries, was fascinating.

One of my favorite attendings was an old-fashioned trauma surgeon who had thirty-five years of experience and had even served in Vietnam, where he had performed surgery in tents. Dr. Seibel was the director of trauma at our trauma center, which had an unusually high number of patients with penetrating traumas—those who had sustained injuries like gunshots and stabbings. He was credited with once joking about the "God complex" so many people and movies assign to surgeons: "We're not playing God by any means," he said. "We're simply giving God a chance to change his mind." He was a true surgeon in every sense of the meaning. He came from an era that was special. I consider myself extremely lucky to have trained under him, an experience I believe is deeply missed in today's surgical training programs.

During my general surgery residency, I met a very cool private-practice plastic surgeon, Dr. Ray Schultz, who was open to letting residents shadow him. The more I learned about what he did, the more interested I became. Plastic surgery is one of the last fields in surgery that treats the whole body. It is performed on all areas of the body and includes cosmetic plastic and trauma facial surgeries, head and neck surgeries, reconstruction of the chest and arms following cancer treatment, hand surgeries, craniofacial surgeries, and more. A plastic surgery fellowship requires an additional two years of training, so for that, I came to Charleston, South Carolina, and upon completion of the training, I was hired to be a faculty member at MUSC. There, I performed a lot of reconstruction procedures, mainly for breast cancer patients, specifically utilizing microsurgery techniques. I also founded and directed the Advanced Breast Reconstruction Program at the National Cancer Institute–designated Hollings Cancer Center.

After about five years in practice, I fulfilled a long-term goal, one I had talked about for years, which was pursuing an MBA. I enrolled at the Darla Moore School of Business at the University of South Carolina, where I completed a master's in business administration with a concentration in international business. I then transitioned into private practice, where I focus primarily on cosmetic plastic surgery of the face and body. Today, my practice, Sweetgrass Plastic Surgery, has grown to multiple offices in the Charleston area, including in Daniel Island, Kiawah Island, Summerville, and West Ashley.

One of the most fulfilling aspects of my job is the positive impact it can have on patients and their family. I saw that quite often when doing cancer reconstructions. I was with patients as they went from uncertainty and fear when initially diagnosed all the way through the reconstruction itself. Often, they were fairly young women with families, and it commonly took a year or more for them to go through surgery, followed by chemotherapy or radiation, and then rehabilitation and reconstruction. In all that, the patients most often looked forward to reconstruction, which was a sort of closure for them that allowed them to get on with their lives.

The truth is that plastic surgery is often undervalued, both in academia and in other medical fields. It is not viewed as true medicine or surgery and often joked about as not being real surgery. Ironically, it is one of the most competitive medical training programs to be accepted into out of medical school. What sets it apart is its ability to have a life-altering effect on patients, to help them really refocus and enjoy their lives and feel more confident about themselves. No other surgical field has the ability that plastic surgery has to help people fix things that affect their self-confidence and can really impact their family lives and relationships. In addition, patients often have the highest expectations—at times, unrealistic expectations—because it is elective and not covered by insurance, so they pay for the procedures themselves. Plastic surgery patients can be some of the most demanding and difficult patients to manage in medicine.

People seek out plastic surgery for reasons that are very real to them, even though others may not see them as important. Sometimes people need to do what matters to them, regardless of what others think. I found that out when I was in college. I went on a basketball scholarship. I was the first in my family to seriously pursue an upper-level education. Still, it came as quite a surprise to some members of my family when I chose to enter medical school. Since no one else in our family had attempted education or a career of that magnitude, there were some naysayers who thought I should just get through college playing sports and then get a job. My father wasn't one of them. He is nicknamed "the General" and is the most happy-go-lucky person I've ever known, always with a kind word to say. Although he did not go to college, he wanted me to get a good education and use it to take me as far as possible. As a father myself, I now realize that seeing your children happy and successful and becoming good people is the greatest joy a person can know. I have one desire for all my children, and that is for them to find their happiness, embrace it, and simply enjoy their lives.

Once I found medicine, I was determined to see it through. I was driven, in part, by the experience of witnessing my mother battle brain cancer, which ultimately took her life in her forties. In dealing with her declining health, I was pretty heavily exposed to medicine from the perspective of a patient's relative, and since she died weeks before I started medical school, I entered medicine from that perspective, which I've tried to maintain throughout my medical career. It has helped me treat patients more as I would treat my own family, instead of talking down to them or making them feel uncomfortable. I have compassion for what they are going through, and I listen to them and their concerns, along with the concerns of their family members. On those highly active days when the chaos of a busy practice can get a little frustrating, I try to feel what the patient and the patient's family are feeling, and my effort to empathize with the patient and patient's family hopefully helps make my patient's experience the best it can be. While my office staff and I practice cosmetic plastic surgery every day, for a patient, the hour they are in our office may be their only experience. They are naturally hesitant, intimidated, and oftentimes outright embarrassed to be there in the first place discussing their deepest insecurities. It is our responsibility to make their experience the best we possibly can and make them feel comfortable.

So my education, combined with my professional training and determination to be compassionate toward patients, has motivated my success in private practice.

And now I want to share my insights into plastic surgery. I wrote this book partly out of my own frustrations but also to help dispel many of the myths and misunderstandings about plastic surgery, a subject that can be very intimidating for a lot of people. I want to help people better understand plastic surgery and decide whether they are good candidates for surgery. Ultimately, I want to help make the overall experience better for anyone considering plastic surgery. It is often said that the hardest part of any surgeon's training is not learning how to do the procedures themselves, but learning whom not to operate on. Ultimately, the combination of a motivated, realistic, and informed patient—and a reasonable, experienced surgeon— hopefully translates to high-quality outcomes and happy, satisfied patients. My hope is that this book serves as a tool in helping you along your journey to finding inner beauty.

One way to help you gain a better understanding is by first clarifying the difference between plastic surgery and cosmetic surgery. Cosmetic surgery is restoration or improvement in appearance only, not dealing with function, while plastic surgery is the return of form and function, which includes cosmetic surgery as a major component of training and practice. Most people see no real difference between cosmetic and plastic surgery. But the medical profession sees a great deal of difference, including training and certification. Board certification by the American Board of Plastic Surgery requires additional training, which can

> Cosmetic surgery is restoration or improvement in appearance only, not dealing with function.

either be two or three more years of plastic surgery beyond training in general surgery, or it can be five or six years of training solely in plastic surgery. Cosmetic surgery is part of the required training for plastic surgeons, but it is not a specialty recognized by the American Board of Medical Specialists (ABMS). Any medical doctor can claim to be a cosmetic doctor, but only surgeons who have completed the ABMS-approved training program in plastic surgery are considered plastic surgeons. I am board certified by the American Board of Plastic Surgery, which is an ABMS-recognized board. I am also a fellow of the American College of Surgeons (FACS). When choosing a plastic surgeon, look for one who has hospital privileges. In order to perform procedures in the hospital, a surgeon must go before a credentialing board to ensure they are adequately trained and certified to hold privileges to perform given procedures. A cosmetic "board-certified" surgeon would not achieve credentialing by a hospital for cosmetic procedures. Some cosmetic surgeons work only in an office setting and do not have privileges to perform cosmetic surgery procedures in a hospital setting. That can be an important factor for the more invasive procedures.

By sharing some insider insights, I hope to dispel many of the myths and misunderstandings that people have about plastic surgery. Most of all, my hope is to improve patients' overall experience with plastic surgery and to let them know there are other folks out there who have similar concerns, experiences, and questions.

As a plastic surgeon, I help women and men, from teens to seniors. Procedures range from breast enhancement to body contouring to facial surgery. They include everything from breast augmentation or reduction to tummy tucks and neck lifts to rhinoplasty (nose jobs) and blepharoplasty (eye lifts). I also do liposuction and fat grafting to all areas of the body. And I offer a whole array of noninvasive laser therapies and injectable products, such as fillers and neurotoxins like Botox.

In the pages ahead, I've included a number of real-life stories but have changed the names of patients to protect their privacy. I am sharing these stories in part to help you get a better sense of the type of personality that does well with plastic surgery. It is important to understand early on that plastic surgery is an art. Dealing with changes in body tissue is not an exact science. Unfortunately, there are no guarantees. So before undergoing any plastic surgery procedure, it is important to understand that it is a process. And while everything can be put exactly in place during surgery, healing is an entirely different piece in the process. The body changes over time, and alterations or revisions may need to be made after healing.

The key to successful plastic surgery is to build a relationship of trust with the plastic surgeon. That can help ensure good communication throughout the process. The more you know about the process itself early on, the better the experience you're going to have. In fact, I tell patients that "I cannot promise perfect outcomes or 100 percent satisfaction with every single procedure. But I will stick with you and do everything possible to ensure that, in the end, you are happy and satisfied, whatever that may take to achieve."

This book was written to provide a strong foundation for anyone considering plastic surgery. I believe the more information you have as a potential patient, a current patient, or a patient's family member, the more enjoyable your experience will be. Hopefully, you will be happy with your plastic surgery procedure, its outcome, and the overall impact it has on your life. When used in the right manner, cosmetic plastic surgery can help you find your beauty.

"BEAUTY IS NOT IN
THE FACE; BEAUTY IS A
LIGHT IN THE HEART."

—KAHLIL GIBRAN

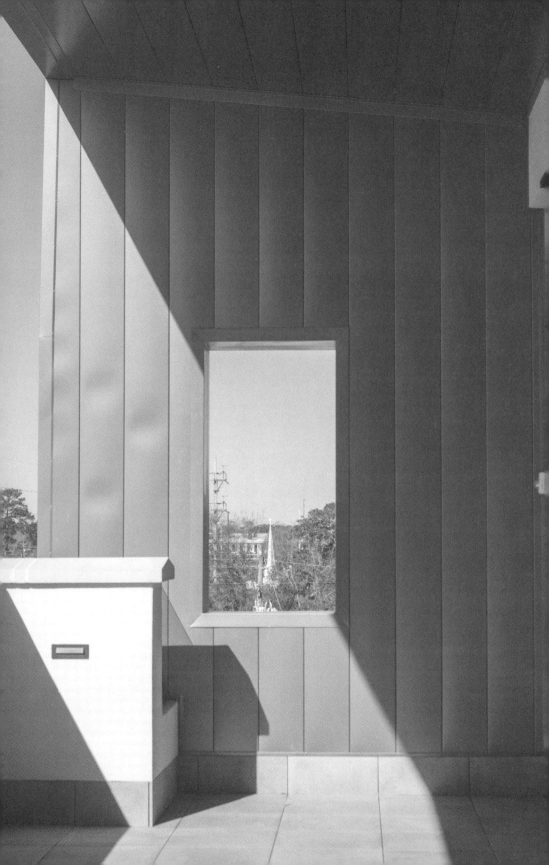

CHAPTER 1

"I Can't Believe I'm Actually Here"

AM I BEING VAIN?

What's the first thing someone says when they try an outfit on or are finished getting ready for a night out? *How do I look? What do you think?* In short, appearance matters. Whether we think it's right or wrong, it transcends basically every part of our life. We make almost every choice based on appearance to some degree. We don't buy clothes or cars that we deem ugly because we always want to look our best. We even choose produce and other foods based on their appearance because we want the best for our bodies. Fruit, produce, cars, clothing, employees, and even technology devices—we automatically and immediately associate a value not only with an item's appearance, but we also allow that bias on appearance to translate to some form or indication of the quality of the item.

It is superficial—most of us know deep down that the association of quality to beauty is not always true. In fact, at times it may even be misleading or flat-out wrong. In other words, the appearance may mislead you into believing that it's a better-quality or better-performing item than it really is. We all do this in all areas of our daily life. To deny that basic fact is to lack insight.

In fact, appearance can be so powerful and influential on one's opinion of another person that attractive people are sometimes viewed as standoffish, too good for everyone else, or not personable. These assumptions are made simply based on their appearance. Several studies point to the ways in which appearance can make a significant difference. More than talent and having the right connections, one study on beauty in the workplace found that well-groomed, attractive people make more money—as much as 12 percent more.[1] In another study, hiring managers were shown photos of attractive and unattractive individuals and asked whether they would hire the person for desirable or less-desirable jobs. In all three experiments, the attractive individuals were more likely to be hired for the more desirable job.[2] In fact, studies have identified what is known as the "halo effect," which is that attractive people are often also perceived as being more intelligent, more successful, wealthier, and so on.[3]

---

1   Daniel Hamermesh, *Beauty Pays: Why Attractive People Are More Successful* (New Jersey: Princeton University Press, 2011), in Daniel Bortz, "Why It Pays to Be Attractive," *U.S. News & World Report*, August 30, 2012, accessed November 22, 2019, https://money.usnews.com/money/personal-finance/articles/2012/08/30/why-it-pays-to-be-attractive.

2   "If you believe attractive people get hired every time, think again," *Economic Times*, October 25, 2017, accessed November 22, 2019, https://economictimes.indiatimes.com/magazines/panache/if-you-believe-attractive-people-get-hired-every-time-think-again/articleshow/61220600.cms.

3   Gregory Ciotti, "The Surprising Power of a Beautiful Face," *Psychology Today*, December 7, 2014, accessed November 22, 2019, https://www.psychologytoday.com/us/blog/habits-not-hacks/201412/the-surprising-power-beautiful-face.

However, a more recent study found that people who are considered "unattractive" may actually earn as much or more than their "attractive" counterparts. Why? The newer study also looked at the role of intelligence, good health, and personality factors—such as being more extroverted, less neurotic, and more open to experiences—concluding that these tend to go hand in hand with good looks.[4] In other words, attractive people don't earn more because of their looks, but because they are also more intelligent, healthier, and have more outgoing and likable personalities.

Initially, while we often think of beauty more in terms of physical attributes, it is also about the emotional connection you have to a person, thing, or circumstance that makes you feel good. The saying "Beauty is only skin deep" is certainly true on some level, but inner beauty is what comes through when someone feels really confident, when they feel more in control.

Simply put, a nice-looking face might get you noticed and help make a good first impression. But it's the way you carry and present yourself that makes you memorable. It's one thing to *look* refreshed; it's another to convey that in your personality—as someone who is confident, friendly, and engaging. The better you feel about yourself on the outside, the better you feel about yourself on the inside—and that inner beauty is what others truly see.

While cosmetic plastic surgery can help you look beautiful on the outside, true beauty comes from embracing your inner self. You can improve your performance in the workplace by feeling better about yourself, whether that's from losing weight, exercising, or having a plastic surgery procedure that makes you feel refreshed. Beauty is

---

4   Satoshi Kanazawa and Mary C. Still, "Is There Really a Beauty Premium or an Ugliness Penalty on Earnings?" *Journal of Business and Psychology*, vol. 33, issue 2 (April 2018), 249–262, accessed November 22, 2019, https://link.springer.com/article/10.1007/s10869-017-9489-6.

basically a feeling of self-confidence that translates into an outer expression of happiness. More people want to be around you, involved with you, and like you or similar to you. That inner beauty outwardly expressed is almost contagious. You can see it when someone enters a room; there are some people who just change the entire dynamic with their presence—ideally for better, but you can see it in people who change the dynamic for worse as well.

Ultimately, it's the outgoingness that increases your performance and success, not just a static picture of how you look in the mirror. Maybe you remember the Dos Equis beer commercials about "the most interesting man in the world"? Notice that they didn't pin that campaign on being "the most attractive." It was more about how the character that was created carried himself: he lived vicariously through himself, had a passport that required no photo, and was so respected the mosquitoes refused to bite him, according to several of the humorous ad messages.[5] What was interesting about the ads is that they went against the typical marketing paradigm in the United States, targeting an emotional connection that wasn't based purely on appearance. I remember talking about the ads in my MBA classes and how the ad agency that created them had taken a poll of people ages twenty-five to thirty-five and found that they placed greater emphasis on being interesting than being attractive—if you were going to sit down and have a beer, it wouldn't matter so much what the person looked like, but how interesting they were.

---

5   Sal Bommarito, "22 of the Best Dos Equis 'The Most Interesting Man in the World' Quotes," *Mic.com*, July 4, 2012, accessed December 7, 2019, https://www.mic.com/articles/9659/22-of-the-best-dos-equis-the-most-interesting-man-in-the-world-quotes-video.

The strategy worked: the campaign helped up the company's sales by 14 percent, according to one spokesman.[6] The campaign ended after a ten-year run because what people find interesting has changed. It's not about what others are doing that's most interesting, but "it's more about standing up for what you think is right and following your passion and your entrepreneurial drive," a company spokesman said in an interview.[7] Marketing must shift with the desires of the consumer—not only of who the consumer is at the time, but more importantly, who they are trying to be or what image they want to portray. Dos Equis had to shift because social norms began to change. Today, social awareness and consciousness are more focused upon by the consumer, and that obviously affects the cosmetic plastic surgery business. What was in style in the 1990s is not the same today.

Still, it happens to nearly everyone—the seconds, minutes, days in life add up until that point when you look in the mirror and do not really like what you see. Many people who want to pursue cosmetic plastic surgery wait, in part because of public perception.

You are constantly on the go—with a job, kids, a life. Responsibilities pile on, and you just do not have the time to take care of yourself. You're running to meetings, eating poorly, traveling for work, taking care of the family. No matter what you eat, no matter how regularly you work out, nothing seems to stop the gradual changes that are occurring to that face in the mirror.

The American culture has long been one that has conditioned people to believe that the desire to look better is all about vanity. There is a perception that taking care of yourself is a bad thing. Even today, when—let's face it—everyone wants to look good, there's a

6   Dale Buss, "A 'Most Interesting' Transition: 5 Questions with André Woldt, Dos Equis," *BrandChannel*, June 14, 2016, accessed December 7, 2019, https://www. brandchannel.com/2016/06/14/5-questions-dos-equis-061416/.

7   Ibid.

stigma attached to plastic surgery, so much so that celebrities who have obviously had a procedure done will deny it, as if it were taboo to be attractive again after good looks have faded. All that stigma does is add to the hurdles that people face regarding their own self-images, something many people struggle with for years. Why shouldn't you have something done if it makes you happier and gives you self-confidence? Think about it: you can improve your performance in the workplace by feeling better about yourself. By being a stronger person on the inside, you can make a bigger impact on the outside. Whether you lose some weight or exercise or have a cosmetic plastic surgery procedure that makes you refreshed, it's really your outgoingness from feeling better about yourself that increases your performance and success—not just that static picture in the mirror.

Who says you can't be both a good person with values and still care about how you look? Of all the things there are to be concerned about in this world, worrying about what others think doesn't seem worthy of the effort and emotional drain. If you're unhappy about a physical feature, and something can be done to make it look better, why worry whether others will think you're being vain? In fact, why do they feel the need to share those negative views—would they do the same if, instead of a facelift, you were buying a bigger house or a Ferrari? Does someone who tells you to "just live with it" really have your best interests in mind? Why should it matter to them, and why does their opinion have a voice in who you are? Are your happiness and self-confidence less important than someone else's opinion of how you should live your life? Will your last thoughts be "I'm glad I did what made others happy," or should they be more along the lines of "I did everything I could to enjoy my life and be the best I could be—for myself and others"?

When it comes to plastic surgery, you must remember that the decisions you make regarding any procedure must be right for you—

and *only you* know what is right for you. That starts by being honest and realistic with yourself. Understanding what is right for you can be difficult since a lot of mystery, misinformation, and social complexity still surround plastic surgery. Although on some levels, it remains a taboo subject—one that people only talk about in whispers—at the same time, it fills the mainstream media.

On any given day, you can find an article about plastic surgery in the news. Most of the reports are not really upbeat. Often it is about a celebrity who has been out of the public eye for a few months and then returns looking different. With everyone fighting for headlines today, it seems that the more drama involved, the more attention the story gets, and the more people tend to buy into what they are reading. That may explain the success of the Kardashian franchise.

But most of the stories are blown out of proportion, or they just do not tell the real story of what happens with the majority of plastic surgery procedures. Think of TV shows such as *Botched* and *Dr. 90210*, which really only represent the extremes. It is a little like flying commercially: airplanes take off and land safely day after day, but the only time they make the news is when something controversial or disastrous happens. With surgery, there are no 100 percents. I can tell you the chances of something happening. But even if that chance is only 1 percent, if it happens to you, then it's 100 percent to you. I cannot underscore this enough: it is crucial with elective surgical procedures to understand that a patient freely chooses to undergo them without any guarantees. If a surgeon is guaranteeing you a surgical outcome, be very careful in choosing them for your procedure.

My hope with this book is to transcend all the chaos, because for most people, plastic surgery is very much like any other surgery. The vast majority of procedures are pretty straightforward, uneventful procedures that produce subtle but real and significant changes. With this book, I hope to draw for you a clearer picture of what plastic surgery is about: what kind of people go in for a plastic surgery procedure, why they do it, and what to expect.

Everyone has a physical feature that bothers them. It may be something they have had since childhood. For women, it may be changes resulting from childbearing. For men and women, it may be the natural body changes that come with aging. Even though they may deny it or downplay it, men are equally worried—or even more worried—about their appearance.

> My hope with this book is to transcend all the chaos, because for most people, plastic surgery is very much like any other surgery.

Regardless of their reason for wanting cosmetic plastic surgery, patients often tell me they are hesitant, reserved, or even embarrassed about having something done. People go for years or decades feeling that everything else is more important than taking care of a feature they dislike about themselves. They try to rationalize their reasons for not doing something about "a little thing" that bothers them because they are embarrassed that it matters to them so much. The reality is that since that "little thing" does bother them, it affects how they carry themselves, and that affects how they're seen by others. It's a vicious circle: they're embarrassed they have a problem, they're embarrassed they're letting it be a problem, and they're embarrassed they're not doing something about it.

People hesitate to pursue plastic surgery, even if it's something minor, because they feel family and friends see their desires as foolish. "Worrying about how I look is trivial compared to everything else," people often think, and they are sure other people feel the same way.

It is true that some people appear to have the perfect life—the perfect house, the perfect family, the perfect figure, the perfect face. Yet often, that person whose life seems "perfect" sees many imperfections in themselves. That can then affect their self-confidence.

Getting over that feeling of selfishness or vanity is a real hurdle for many people. Often, they are so concerned about what other people will think of them if they change their appearance that they forgo having anything done, even though they are dissatisfied with something about themselves. They would rather be unhappy with themselves than feel they're disappointing someone or are being seen as selfish.

In truth, plastic surgery can be a selfless act because it can make people happier and even more productive. Once they do something that achieves their goals, they become more dynamic, more interactive, more social.

How most people perceive themselves and how they look outwardly are two very different views. Not a day goes by that I don't tell a patient, "You are unequivocally your own worst critic." As someone in his midforties with seven children, I can certainly relate to that level of self-perception as I age. Even though I work on people every day, I joke about getting old and looking older all the time, or I at least partially joke about it. But there's no doubt that the face in the mirror is different. I'm starting to look older, and that seemed to happen overnight. My own father—the least vain person in the world—even expressed to me when he was in his sixties that he didn't recognize the person he saw in his reflection. "It's amazing," he said. "I look in the mirror today, and I'm not sure who the person is looking back at me." No matter how good you may feel, or how active you may be, the aging process marches on. My goal is to simply help slow that march. It's bittersweet to hear people say, "I feel so much healthier and active than I look. I look a lot older than I feel." These people have one request: to simply look as good as they feel.

On the other hand, some people know they do not look their best. They see the gradual changes taking place, and they agonize over what they see. But again, they do not do anything about it. Then, a major life event tips the scales and gets them to move from being bothered about a feature to actually doing something about it. A life-changing illness, the long-distance move of a close friend, or the death of a parent or spouse acts as a wake-up call. That's when reality sets in: they realize life is short, and it is time to do something for themselves, something they have always wanted to do. There should be no shame, hesitance, or uncertainty in that. They deserve it.

There are other triggers that get people to undergo plastic surgery. It may be an innocent comment such as "Is that your daughter next to you in that picture?" (It is your sister.) Maybe it is an upcoming reunion. Everyone wants to appear successful when around their former classmates. For many people, whether they were popular in high school or not, the peer pressure remains very real even decades later.

One patient, Kate, came in for some work before her daughter's wedding. Since her daughter had been born when Kate was in her midthirties, the daughter's friends had always referred to Kate as "the old mom" in their social group. Kate finally decided that she did not want to be "the old mom" at her daughter's wedding.

For others, the trigger is about wanting to look and feel better following a perceived failure in life, such as a divorce. Yet other people want plastic surgery to enhance a success in life such as celebrating a new career—a high-level sales position, for instance—that they want to approach with their "best face and body possible."

Moms are especially guilty of putting off doing something for themselves for far too long. Their children, their spouses, even their jobs always come first. They have done so much, for so long, for so many other people that they are uncomfortable about doing something for themselves. But the mom who is so self-conscious about her body that she will not get dressed up and go out to eat with her husband, or won't go to the pool with the kids, or rarely goes out in public at all, may be making her whole family less happy. In America, the culture is one that tends to place women who have had children into a "mom" stereotype, a place where they should no longer be concerned about their looks. The woman's family, friends, and spouse may wonder what she is up to—and why—if she suddenly starts caring about how she looks. That makes it harder for that mother to realize that by doing something for herself, she will be a happier person—her happiness is important to others and makes others happy.

No one wants to feel out of place in a roomful of people. People want to look and feel as if they have great lives. No matter how chaotic their life is, no matter how many children they may have, or how many schedules they have to keep, they want to appear as if they have it all together. For a mom especially, there's no bigger compliment than to see people show surprise when they find out she has four kids. A compliment like that instills people with confidence in how they appear and present themselves. And that carries over into home life, work life, and social life. It can really make a huge difference.

Mothers also want to teach their children, especially their daughters, how to be confident about who they are. They want their children to face the world with confidence—and that starts with their own self-confidence.

Today, it can be more difficult to have that kind of self-confidence and not care about what others think, especially in a world where everyone is constantly being photographed. With the constant posting of selfies and other images on social media websites such as Facebook and Instagram, people are always being made aware of how they look and how their appearances are changing. Patients tell me all the time that they didn't truly grasp their appearance until they saw themselves on their cell phone screen when they turned it on to take a selfie.

Only a few years ago, the only way to recall a wedding, vacation, or other activity was to page through a photo album. Now, on your phone, you can see how you looked an hour ago, a day ago, a week ago. And there's little control over where your photo appears. Anyone who knows you can snap a photo and post it online. You're out there more than you want to be, and you're constantly reminded of how you look and how you're aging and changing. Plus, the pandemic has forced us to stay home and find other ways to communicate. Although technology has allowed us to stay in contact, we are seeing each other on video screens now, which aren't always the most flattering. Right now, I have a patient who is the CEO of a company, and she is trying to raise money on Zoom calls—she's come for some plastic surgery because she knows how important it is for her to look well rested and energetic.

In fact, in 2021, the AAFPRS's annual survey found that 83 percent of providers said their patients were pursuing cosmetic plastic surgery procedures because they wanted to look better on virtual calls.[8] It can be particularly distressing to have a child so worried about their looks simply because of online peer pressure. There are really no age requirements to get an Instagram account, leaving kids subjected to a world that they're really not mature enough to fully understand—a world that's all about appearance. In fact, some sites actually have available "beautification face filters" that users can apply to their image to make

---

8   "AAFPRS Announces Annual Survey Results: A Look at How Covid-19 Disrupted Facial Plastic Surgery & Aesthetics," news release, February 1, 2021, American Academy of Facial Plastic and Reconstructive Surgery, accessed February 24, 2021, https://www.aafprs.org/Media/Press_Releases/New%20Stats%20AAFPRS%20 Annual%20Survey.aspx.

them more like a magazine. In the face of these perceived guidelines of perfection that can subconsciously see themselves as flawed, how does a mom (or dad) looking to cosmetically enhance their own appearance explain to a child that what matters is on the inside?

This is one area where I, as a cosmetic plastic surgeon, often have to draw a line—performing a procedure purely for appearance on a child who is still developing is helping them into a trap of always trying to "fit in." That's creating a dangerous spiral that can leave them perpetually dissatisfied with their own appearance. But I also think it is possible to teach your children that you can have self-confidence in who you are and still want to improve your appearance when doing it for the right reasons. It has to be for you, not to impress friends or try to make other people see you differently.

The reasons people finally decide to pursue cosmetic plastic surgery vary, but three of the most common are these: (1) they finally recognize the need for it, (2) they have the resources to do it because they are financially stable—often that's because they've climbed the corporate ladder and the kids are grown and gone, and (3) they're at a place in life where they are comfortable and confident and don't care what others think.

However, in the region where I practice, the southeastern United States, people are still very conservative. Nobody wants to look "overdone." They want improvement but don't want anything extreme. They often reference one of the many celebrities out there who have overdone it and say, "I don't want that look." In fact, every year, the American Academy of Facial Plastic and Reconstructive Surgery (AAFPRS) surveys its members to look at the top trends. In 2018, the survey found that 41 percent of patients said a "fear of looking unnatural" was their primary concern.[9] Most people simply want to look good for their age. For instance, if they are sixty years old, they want to appear to be a vibrant, healthy, rested sixty-year-old.

As I write this book, there is actually a trend by some younger adults to look for ways to retain their youthful looks longer. The AAFPRS's 2018 survey found that nearly three-fourths of facial plastic surgeons (72 percent) saw an increase in patients under age thirty seeking cosmetic plastic surgery.[10] Surgical procedures were up 47 percent, and Botox injections were up 22 percent since 2013. In 2019, nonsurgical procedures were up another 13 percent, and minimally invasive procedures such as skin treatments, fillers, and neurotoxins/Botox comprised 85 percent of the total number of procedures performed.[11]

The truth is that the decision to have cosmetic plastic surgery should be a decision you make for yourself, even though those around you may benefit. When you look better and feel better about who you are, you are better for other people around you. Plastic surgery can be the first step in turning a corner to becoming a better you. And you don't need anyone else's approval or acceptance to do that.

What's important to recognize is that the definition of happiness can change over time. What matters when you are twenty-three years old may not be the same thing that matters to you at age forty. For example, these days, one of the reasons for plastic surgery is to remove

---

9 "AAFPRS Annual Survey Reveals Key Trends in Facial Plastic Surgery," *American Academy of Facial Plastic and Reconstructive Surgery*, January 23, 2019, news release, accessed November 22, 2019, https://www.aafprs.org/Media/Press_Releases/2019Jan23_AnnualTrendSurveyResults.aspx.

10 Ibid.

11 "New Stats: AAFPRS Annual Survey Reveals Face of Plastic Surgery Goes Younger," news release, February 11, 2020, American Academy of Facial Plastic and Reconstructive Surgery, accessed October 11, 2020, https://www.aafprs.org/Media/Press_Releases/New%20Stats%20AAFPRS%20Annual%20Survey.aspx.

or reduce the size of breast implants in women who had them put in when they were in their twenties, when large breasts were in vogue. But now, these women are forty years old and are miserable because their necks and backs hurt, and their skin is stretched out. Add a few pounds of middle-age weight, and their breasts just look too big for their frames. Many patients tell me, "I don't know what I was thinking." Well, twenty-three-year-old thinking is different from forty-year-old thinking. Just as priorities change, the definition of beauty changes with time. In their twenties, women may want large breasts and a Barbie-doll figure in a swimsuit. In their forties, they just want to be more active, and they don't want neck and back pain from large implants.

I have taken breast implants out of many women who have had them for several years before finally deciding they wanted them removed. They didn't replace the implants; they simply wanted them out. Since it's fairly common for older women to have their larger implants replaced with smaller ones, I thought initially that patients asking to have theirs removed and not replaced with smaller ones would surely be unhappy with that decision, and I explained that to them during the consultation before the procedure. However, to date, not one of them has asked to have the implants replaced. Every one of them says they feel better physically, and they feel better about themselves. In some ways, putting the implants in when they were young was about fitting a perceived image. Now, years later, taking the implants out is simply about their own self-happiness. They have grown into being content with who they are and what is most comfortable or practical. They are no longer concerned with impressing someone else. In a way, they have come full circle.

When it comes to men, especially older men, they also are often uncomfortable with the idea of plastic surgery. For them, being concerned about their appearance is not "manly." They are probably as insecure—or more insecure—about their appearance as any woman might be, but they project, or try to project, confidence in, or indifference to, their appearance. The truth is that men face the same body-change challenges as women do, and they care about how they look just as much as women do. In reality, as I mentioned earlier, perception and opinions matter to men maybe even more than to women. When it comes to stereotypes and critics, a man's situation may be worse: society is even slower to embrace men's desires to improve how they look. That inner turmoil can be very difficult for men.

Men do not want to talk about their defects. They do not want to point out anything that could be seen as a weakness or flaw. They don't want to appear vulnerable. And they are notorious for not wanting to ask for help.

Men who do choose to explore the possibility of undergoing plastic surgery seem to be especially embarrassed when they come into my office. Often, a man will come in with his wife, who will talk about herself first and then open up the conversation to what he's considering having done—almost as if it's an afterthought. It is hard for some men to talk about themselves in front of the women who staff my practice. Sometimes it's a generational issue. Men who are part of the baby boomer generation often worked in jobs involving physical labor. They did not necessarily worry about how they looked because that did not matter on the job.

We live in a different world today. Men are more concerned with their appearance: their hair, their clothes, their overall looks. Today it is more acceptable for men to publicly talk about looks. Every day, there's a new product on the market for men who want to change the way they look.

So men are coming in for cosmetic plastic procedures these days, especially with technology that allows for less-invasive procedures. Men are looking for procedures that deliver more subtle changes with quick recoveries because they want work done "under the radar" essentially. They don't want others to know they've had something done because of what they believe others will think. As a result, when they do show up, it's usually because they've put off doing something for themselves for many years, just as women do.

Plastic surgery is beginning to be a viable option for two reasons: (1) it is a way to take care of something about yourself that has been on your mind, and (2) photo sharing and social media are opening possibilities for people who might not have considered them in the past. For instance, when someone sees how good Aunt Betty looks year after year, they want to know how she does it—and plastic surgery may well be that *how*. Plastic surgery has become more accessible, goals are attainable, and the internet has made the process of finding a plastic surgeon simpler.

Rarely does one procedure dramatically change every aspect of a person's life, and anyone going into the process with that attitude is likely to be sorely disappointed. The situation is similar to marketing in the United States, where magazine photos showing a tall, beautiful woman with a perfect body, a nice car, a phenomenal house, and the perfect mate would have you believe that getting one of those things automatically means you'll have all the others. Of course she's smiling! She's got the perfect life! Those kinds of images can lead people to believe that changing one feature means everything else will automatically be different. Young girls, for instance, often believe that bigger breasts can lead to an ideal lifestyle, the perfect mate, the perfect job, and more. Bigger breasts can help a woman fit better into a swimming suit, but they won't automatically give her a picture-perfect life. Yes, areas of her life may change, but that will be the result of her own change of mindset, including improved self-confidence. With the right attitude, she may overcome life's hurdles (including self-doubts from all those whispers of "What has she had done?").

Studies have found that people whose expectations are in line with realistic outcomes usually feel that plastic surgery can significantly boost confidence. In fact, in a European study, a majority of respondents reported feeling a boost in their self-confidence and greater enjoyment in life after undergoing plastic surgery. In the study, only 12 percent of respondents had higher expectations that the surgery would do the impossible for them. Of the 550 people surveyed, 87 percent of whom were women, most said they "felt healthier, were less anxious, had developed more self-esteem and found the operated body feature in particular, but also their body as a whole, more attractive."[12] If you feel more attractive, does it matter what critics think?

Again, the bottom line is that it is not about what other people think; it is about what's best for you. Cosmetic plastic surgery is about being honest with yourself. It is not about trying to fit into what other people think or what you perceive others to be thinking. It is about what really matters to you. While you may not be a mom who raises people's eyebrows when others hear you have four kids, it is OK to not want to be an "old mom." Happiness matters. It's OK to want to feel self-confident and happy. Anyone who says otherwise is being shallow, judgmental, and oftentimes insecure.

> It is not about what other people think; it is about what's best for you.

---

12   "Plastic Surgery Boosts Happiness, Self-Esteem for Those without 'Unreasonable' Expectations," *New York Daily News*, March 12, 2013, accessed April 24, 2017, http://www.nydailynews.com/life-style/health/plastic-surgery-boosts-happiness-unreasonable-expectations-article-1.1286078.

People are going to think what they are going to think, and those who are the most critical of others often have many issues themselves. If you try to do for yourself only what someone else thinks is reasonable, you're not going to be happy. At some point, you have to decide that what matters is whether the procedure is right for you. After that, it's the role of the plastic surgeon to determine whether plastic surgery can deliver the expected results. The plastic surgeon's job is first and foremost to keep patients safe and then to identify what the patients see as problems and match procedures or treatments to address those issues. We are only successful when patients are safe and happy and their expectations are met.

The procedure doesn't have to be dramatic to make a difference. It can be something simple that produces a subtle change. It can be a combination of several small procedures that can have a cumulative result, require less recovery, and result in overall improved patient satisfaction.

Changing technologies and advances have made all kinds of procedures available today. With the right mindset going in, even a small change can be a big confidence booster. When you start on a journey in search of beauty, the combination of cosmetic plastic surgery and the desire to achieve happiness can deliver a true and lasting inner beauty. Nothing else can truly do that for you.

"IT TAKES NOTHING
TO JOIN THE CROWD.
IT TAKES EVERYTHING
TO STAND ALONE."

—HANS F. HANSEN

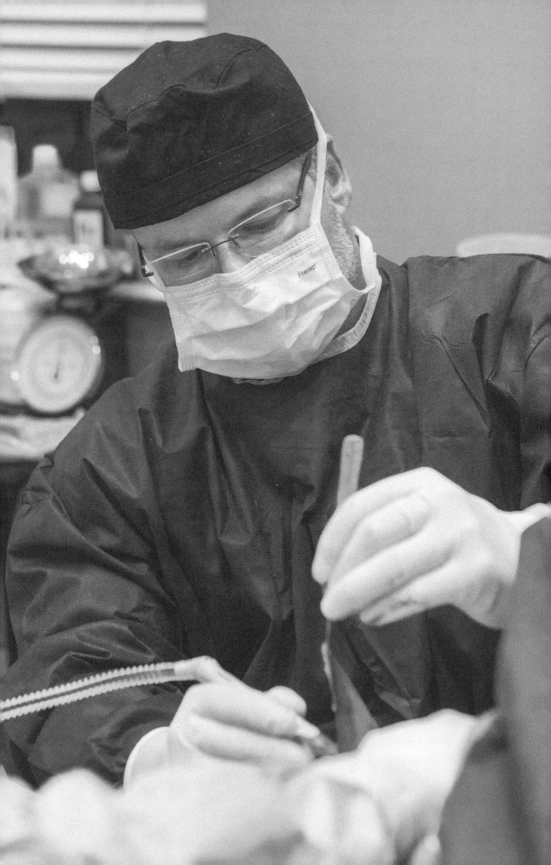

CHAPTER 2

"I Just Want to Be More Like Myself"

I DON'T FEEL LIKE I LOOK.

In her twenties, Eve was healthy and active. While in college, she had participated in competitive sports, and she had always prided herself on being able to wear anything without worry, including a bikini when she went to the beach. Then Eve got married, had three children, and fell into the routine of working from 8:00 a.m. to 5:00 p.m. and taking care of her family.

While she had been able to keep up a reduced exercise routine after having her first child, which allowed her to regain her figure fairly quickly postpregnancy, returning to her healthier lifestyle was a little more challenging after her second child was born. After her third child, Eve was so busy working and taking care of family that having any sort of exercise routine was out of the question. As she launched fully into "mother mode," she found herself choosing fewer healthy foods because she and her family were always on the run. As the children grew into their teens, Eve's unhealthy lifestyle was compounded by declining hormones as perimenopause set in, a scenario that I'm sure sounds all too familiar to many middle-aged women.

Finally, when the last child left for college, when Eve was in her early forties, she decided she needed a change. She committed herself to working out regularly and to fixing healthier meals for herself and her husband.

After losing one hundred pounds, she felt great. She was in a better place physically and emotionally. But as is the case with many people who have lived with their larger selves for so long, Eve was left with excess skin. "I don't look like I feel. In fact, I don't even look like myself. I feel healthy and vibrant, yet I look old," people often tell me when they come in looking for options. That's what Eve told me as well.

What happened to Eve is typical for many women. While other people may view them as healthier—their clothes fit better, they move better, they look happier—these women still see their former selves when they look in the mirror. Instead of seeing someone who has reached a significant health goal, all they see is sagging skin or lack of muscle tone. Women who lose even ten or twenty pounds and are getting regular exercise will say they feel great but will also notice how they look older due to loose, sagging skin. And sagging skin is even more common with significant weight loss. Unfortunately, no diet or exercise program will fix loose, sagging skin. People cannot fix this on their own.

When that happens, they often look to plastic surgery for skin removal and body contouring procedures. And of these people who come in for a procedure, the most satisfied are those with realistic expectations about what plastic surgery can do for them.

They know that the images in today's glamour magazines are often not realistic; those photos have been manipulated. Even some of the cover models don't look like their pictures in real life. The message in today's media puts unrealistic pressure on people, who then place unrealistic pressure on themselves. Female celebrities who have children are often back to modeling or being on camera within three months without looking as if their body ever changed—but that's crazy. Obviously, that's not realistic for most people who don't have the means to employ a personal trainer, a nanny, a chef, and everything else they need to devote all their time to getting their former selves back.

Unrealistic media pressure includes criticizing those who try to improve their looks with plastic surgery for not being natural. Basically, it's a lose-lose situation. The media gives people unrealistic expectations of how they should appear, and people then attempt to meet those unrealistic expectations through plastic surgery—for instance, by doing surgery to reverse aging and childbirth marks. Yet when people try to meet unrealistic expectations through plastic surgery, they're criticized for "having work done" or for not just being happy with who they are and how they look.

Skin removal following significant weight loss requires pursuing plastic surgery for the right reasons. Getting back to a healthy weight can certainly lead to a better lifestyle and a longer, healthier life. Weight has a more dramatic impact on your long-term health than almost anything else, even smoking. It affects your life expectancy and health outcomes more than anything.

But the desire to have plastic surgery to remove sagging skin comes from a different mindset; it is not as much about health as it is about mental outlook. It is crucial to understand that scarring will occur with a skin removal procedure. However, most people who pursue it are not concerned about the scarring. Their main concern is to remove the extra tissue so that their clothes fit better and they can reduce the moisture, rash, and irritation that comes with unwanted skin folds. Having excess skin removed is often the end goal in their weight-loss journey and their attempt to feel better about themselves.

> It is crucial to understand that scarring will occur with a skin removal procedure.

Often, prior to excess-skin excision, patients who have lost weight tell me, "Although it may sound crazy, I still see myself as fat." They don't feel as if they've truly lost the weight, although the scale says differently. When they stand in front of the mirror and see all the excess skin, it just reminds them of who and how they were. The cosmetic plastic surgery portion of their journey gives them closure; it is crucial to making them feel better and more complete.

Still, since a part of the process involves scarring, the process of plastic surgery should include the patient's partner or significant other. The subject of scarring is very real and needs to be addressed up front because once it happens, there's no going back.

Patients who are significantly concerned about scarring must resolve that within themselves before undergoing the procedure. Scarring is a given; every procedure will produce some type of scar. The degree of scarring can be due to all kinds of things, including genetics, the actual healing process, the specific procedure being done, how much pressure or tension there is on the incision or wound, and the location on the body. Age can also play a role in how much scarring the surgery produces. Children's bodies tend to have extremely "revved-up" scars, while older people tend to have less aggressive scarring. I used to perform a number of cleft lip and palate surgeries on children, and their scars can be very red and raised due to their immune and inflammatory response being aggressive, so how they look immediately following surgery is not how they're going to look twelve to eighteen months after the surgery as the red color fades and the scar matures.

Comparing scars is irrelevant; even if your best friend has the same procedure, you will each experience a dramatically different level of scarring. With some procedures and in some individuals, of course, the scarring is less visible, but the severity of most scars will change dramatically over time, and many scars can be improved with subsequent treatment. That takes time, however, so patience is very important when it comes to improving a scar. Otherwise, the revision is being made to skin that is still changing. Without waiting and addressing a scar at the proper time, you're basically starting the whole procedure all over again. I'll discuss the actual healing process in more depth in chapter 7.

Even though many people place all their trust in the plastic surgeon to perform a procedure without leaving a scar, their faith is misguided; no plastic surgeons can, nor should they, guarantee there will be no scarring. All full-thickness incisions or traumatic cuts to the skin will result in scars. All. The degree of scarring is affected by many factors, some of which are out of the plastic surgeon's control, including genetics, skin tone, the location of the scar, and the past tendency to create a degree of scar. Surgical technique, while crucial to overall outcome, plays a less significant role in overall scarring than most patients would guess.

The more realistic your expectations, the better your outcomes when it comes to plastic surgery. As I mentioned earlier, magazines are trying to portray an ideal life and look, the ultimate happiness, and they're associating their message with something they want you to

> All full-thickness incisions or traumatic cuts to the skin will result in scars. All.

think you need. They are selling hope. That message carries over to plastic surgery when patients believe that by looking more like the person in the advertisement, they will also have the idyllic life that advertisement portrays. If you're looking at magazine images and hoping to be something you never were, then your expectations will likely never be met—irrespective of the surgeon, the procedure, or the amount of money you spend.

Now, patients often come in with photos of themselves to show how they used to look. They may have had fuller lips or shapelier legs, and they want to address that feature in the hope of returning to that youthful time in their life. Not only are they looking to physically turn back the clock, but in doing so, they are, to some degree, looking to mentally or emotionally gain back some of their more youthful outlook. The look is associated with a different time in their life, a time when they had no responsibilities, a time before they felt worn out by life. Now that they have it all—the house, the cars, the kids, the financial stability—they want to also regain the youthful energy, appearance, and outlook they once had, and they think plastic surgery will do that for them.

In cases like these, it is up to the plastic surgeon to convey to patients what their results are likely to be. Can the surgeon realistically expect to help a person gain back some of what has changed over time? My role as a plastic surgeon is not to tell patients what they should or shouldn't do but to listen to them and hear what they want changed and how they want it changed. Then, using my experience and expertise, I must determine whether the procedure is going to be safe and in their best interests, and whether it—or another procedure—is going to give them the result they desire. If what they are asking for cannot be done, if their goal is not achievable, if their expectations cannot be met, then they will not be happy with cosmetic plastic surgery. In addition, they will have spent time and money and still have a permanent scar.

Take making lips plumper, for example, which requires a procedure known as lip augmentation. Many older women find themselves with thinner lips than they had when they were younger. Loss of lip volume is a normal part of aging. However, there are a number of ways to replace some of that youthful fullness. For instance, there are new implants that make it easier to achieve great results. Fillers, on the other hand, can be difficult and subjective. That's largely because people have very different views of how much filler makes for the best look. Most people have seen a picture of someone with ducklike lips following an injection. Yet some people with very full lips want still more filler only a couple of weeks after their procedure. In the southeastern area of the United States, where, as I mentioned, people tend to be more conservative, most patients have a small amount of filler just to try out the procedure. If they like their results, they will go back for more. The underlying concern with many of my patients is that they don't want to be "overdone." That is the best way to approach such a procedure. In fact, I tend to be conservative. I would rather add less filler and then touch up the procedure, as needed.

So while people often say, "I just want to be myself," those who will be happiest with their outcomes are the ones who add, "I know I won't look exactly like I did before." That goes with all procedures, from skin removal to tummy tucks to chin lifts to skin peels. Expectations of the patient have to be clearly understood by both the surgeon and, more importantly, the patient themselves. Misalignment of expectations with results is the single biggest cause of discontent by patients having cosmetic plastic surgery.

This is why the first step when consulting a plastic surgeon is to talk about goals and expectations. The surgeon should ask you what you want to get out of your plastic surgery experience. I often will ask the patient to tell me simply, if they were to have the procedure we are considering, what type of outcome will make them happy twelve months from now. The answer to that question is crucial for the plastic surgeon to determine which procedure to use, what kind of outcomes to expect, and whether he or she can help you understand what lies ahead for you. For instance, if a sixty-year-old woman wants to look as she did at twenty years of age or before having kids, the plastic surgeon needs to pause and discuss what the patient really wants in the way of outcomes. What can she realistically expect?

The same goes for patients who say, "Oh, I just want to look better," or "I want to look as good as I feel." It is up to the plastic surgeon to take the time to really drill down and try to get specific about the patient's needs and wants.

For instance, if a forty-year-old woman says she wants to look a little more like she did before she had kids, that is a generally achievable goal in most patients. We can return some of the breast volume she may have lost while lifting and repositioning the breast to a more desirable position. We can help tighten some of the stretched or loose skin in her abdomen as well as tighten the rectus muscle diastasis that occurs, giving her a dramatically improved, flattened abdomen. Those kinds of procedures will deliver realistic results.

However, it is not realistic for a forty-year-old woman, after bearing three children, gaining considerable weight, and getting out of shape, to expect plastic surgery to turn her into a supermodel. If a woman brings in a *Vogue* magazine and says she wants to look like the five-foot-eleven-inch Czechoslovakian supermodel on the cover, it goes without saying, that is not going to happen. In a case like that, chances are there are few procedures that will make that patient truly happy. There are few things a plastic surgeon can do that will help her have a realistic perception of herself. Remember that *Vogue* is a perception. Its advertisements use perfect pictures of flawless models in extraordinarily beautiful surroundings to make you feel an attachment to the advertised product. Those perfect images have been photoshopped or altered to project an ideal image. Ironically, while you may see and think beauty when looking at those photos, getting those photos to make you feel beauty often has the opposite effect.

The reality is that plastic surgery of the face and neck can turn back the clock seven to ten years, on average, depending on the patient's needs, the procedure, and the circumstances. Genetics can determine even better outcomes for some people. For instance, a sixty-five-year-old patient of mine, Mona, who had a neck and lower face lift, told me she sometimes asked people to guess her age, and most of them thought she was in her mid-to-late forties. Naturally, she was extremely happy with her results.

The nose is one example of an area of the face that is subject to the misperceptions that come with plastic surgery. The nose is probably the most deeply analyzed structure on the face, and people's perceptions of noses are extremely varied and individualized. It is ironic that many people say they hate their nose, but when shown a picture of it on its own, they will say what they are seeing is a fine nose. It is a difficult structure to operate on; in many ways it is a situation where literally a millimeter or two matters tremendously. Patients will hyperanalyze their noses to a level that virtually no one else would ever notice.

The nose is one of the obsessions of people who have body dysmorphic disorder, a condition in which dissatisfaction with a physical flaw—real or imagined—develops into an obsession that disrupts daily life. People with this disorder will never be happy with any change, and there is nothing a plastic surgeon can do to remedy the situation. In fact, plastic surgeons are taught in medical school to beware of patients demonstrating the traits identified by the abbreviation SIMON (single, immature, male, overexpectant, and narcissistic). These are men who overvalue rhinoplasty outcomes.

There are two approaches to cosmetic plastic surgery. The first is to make small, gradual changes through multiple sessions. The second approach is to perform multiple surgical procedures in one session. Some folks prefer gradual changes, while others prefer a more dramatic, instantaneous change with one recovery. The crucial point here is to match patients' expectations and goals with the approach that best serves them and, in the end, delivers their best personalized outcome. Depending on the patient's personality, one approach may fit them better than the other. In general, I have found that for those unsure of the process, it is often best to start with smaller, less complex procedures and see the results prior to undergoing further procedures. These patients are the most likely to have good results and to feel that bit of a boost to their confidence may be enough to make them want to try more. By making gradual changes, they know they can, over time, transform into earlier, more youthful versions of themselves.

In addition, the slow, step-wise approach allows the patient and surgeon—and family skeptics—to build a lasting and trusting relationship. Admittedly, some patients have time or other constraints that make it more difficult to have multiple procedures done over time instead of all at once. But again, spacing out the procedures can help build rapport between surgeon and patient, which can ultimately help to better align expectations.

One of my patients, Jennifer, a psychotherapist, was in her sixties when she first came in for some procedures. In the beginning, her husband, Jim, a psychologist, was adamantly against her having anything done. So she started small, with a few skin-care procedures.

In time, she had her eyelids done, and then she had a couple of liposuction procedures. Having work done in increments made Jim more trusting and fully supportive of the process because he'd seen the gradual but significant impact it had on Jennifer and her happiness.

You don't have to get a full-body overhaul when there are many smaller procedures these days that will produce subtle changes. Often, the best candidates are those like Jennifer who want to subtly turn back the clock. They do not want to roll into work after three weeks off and be unrecognizable. They are doing it for themselves, not to impress other people. With that kind of motivation, plastic surgery can achieve lasting and real results.

"THE TRUE BEAUTY
IN A WOMAN IS
REFLECTED IN
HER SOUL."

—AUDREY HEPBURN

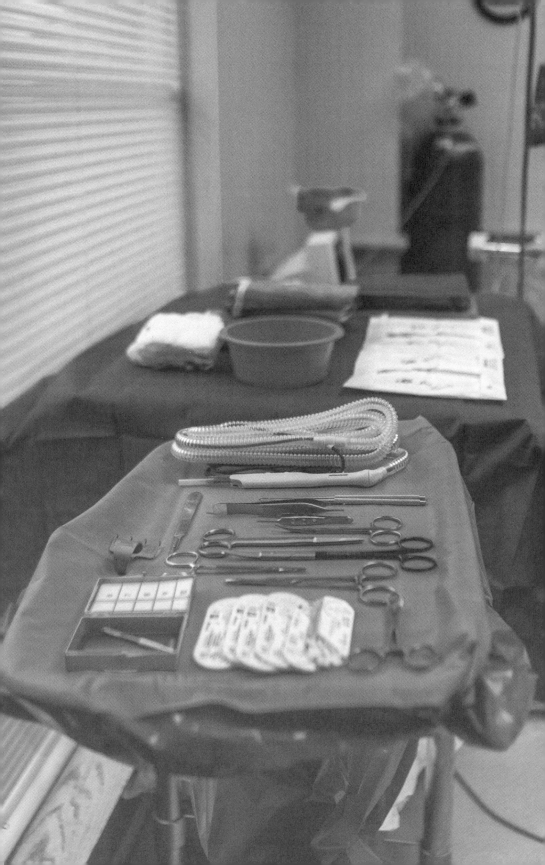

CHAPTER 3

"I Look Older than My Age"

WHAT CAN BE DONE TO REVERSE THIS?

I n her midfifties, Carol woke up one morning and saw in the mirror someone she didn't recognize. "Funny, I don't feel old and tired, but I sure look it," she thought. Carol had an active lifestyle. She regularly walked or worked out with friends, and ate a healthy diet largely of fresh and organic foods.

Still, the face she saw in the mirror was one that belied her age—and not in a good way. All that healthy living made her feel great on the inside, but on the outside, the years had taken their toll. She was looking for a way to turn back the clock, to make her face more closely reflect the strength, spirit, and energy she still felt inside. After all, she knew that's what had helped her succeed in her sales career, but she also felt that it was getting tougher to get a foot in the door just to make her pitch—and that her age was a factor. It was quickly becoming less about her knowledge and accomplishments and more about how she looked. Fair or not, the social perception of aging in men and women is very different. Especially in certain industries, aging is sometimes perceived as a good thing for men, but women are often—unfairly—judged differently.

Still, both women and men ages forty-five to sixty-five really start to notice a difference in their skin when they look in the mirror. Forty-five-year-old skin is healthier than sixty-five-year-old skin, but even at that age, there are less-invasive treatments that can stave off some of the effects of aging.

There are four factors that determine the appearance of aging of the face.

The first factor is the overall healthiness of the skin. Age spots, environmental wear or sun damage, dark discolorations, larger pores, and a loss of shine or vibrancy can add years to a face.

The second factor is the soft-tissue structures, the outer skin and the subcutaneous tissue (the tissue under the skin). Faces that look older have lost subcutaneous tissue for a couple of reasons. One is as a natural part of aging. As people age, that subcutaneous fat diminishes, and patients lose facial volume. The roundness of the face that determines its youthful appearance slowly thins and elongates. The other is lifestyle—activity and dieting can cause a loss of subcutaneous tissue. It's very evident in people who exercise a lot, particularly people who take up running. They tend to have faces that are very drawn, very sunken in. It's the same in people who lose a lot of weight. They feel a lot better after the weight is gone, and they're usually a lot healthier. But when they look in the mirror, they look much older. That's because they've lost subcutaneous tissue.

Once the underlying tissue is gone, the outer layer of skin begins to sag. As the tissue sags on the face, the neck skin loosens and descends. The levels of good collagen and elastin decrease as we age, preventing the skin from being able to tighten. Very thin patients develop neck bands with the loose skin, which can be difficult to treat. Patients who are heavier tend to develop full, loose, sagging necks with both excess fat as well as skin. In addition, the platysma muscles of the neck separate, leading to the "sling" effect under the neck, causing the tissue to loosen and hang as opposed to having a sharp, tight neckline. There are a whole range of treatments to help with a sagging neckline, from noninvasive CoolSculpting, Kybella, and other injectables, to minimally invasive, energy-assisted liposuction, to more definitive surgical treatments like a neck lift to tighten the muscles, lift the soft tissue, and repair the muscle separation. Each patient may present a combination of these clinical problems and thus need an individually tailored treatment approach.

The third factor that affects an aging face is the underlying bone structures. The bone structures of the face lose volume. The cheeks resorb, the chin shrinks, and the underlying cartilage of the nose changes—all add to the aging process. With aging, the bone structure in the face undergoes resorption or loss of volume. It's similar to osteoporosis in other areas of the body, in which bone begins to deteriorate.

The fourth factor is loss of lip volume. As the lips grow thinner, the vertical wrinkles around the lips get deeper.

These changes all age the face. The soft tissue is dropping due to gravity; it's losing volume due to aging; the bone underneath, which holds the soft tissue up, is decreasing in volume or undergoing resorption; and the lips are growing thinner. The tissue and bone changes create more of an upright triangle, with the wider base of the triangle at the jawline. Instead of an inverted triangle from the eyes down to the chin, with the cheekbones wider and the chin narrower, the triangle uprights as a person ages. That's the difference between an aging appearance versus a youthful appearance. When we work on the bone structures, we're trying to recreate the inverted triangle by making the upper portion wider and fuller to lift the tissues to some degree but to also give the appearance that the lower part of the face is thinner.

Depending on the patient's needs and wants, their concerns can be addressed with one or more skin-resurfacing options. These are good, affordable options that have little or no downtime. And they work on multiple areas of the body in addition to the face.

Some of the ways to turn back the clock include the following:

Skin-Care Products

Perhaps because women are more acutely aware of the effects of aging, they have often spent a lifetime on things such as basic skin care. Men, however, tend to not pay attention to their skin for years, and they—sometimes more so than women—tend to have sun damage.

Reversing the aging of the face starts by choosing good skin-care products—and using them. Sunblock is one of the best defenses against the rays that can really age the skin. These are best used early in life to prevent the damage. Good skin care can build a solid foundation, so start skin care before spending money on other efforts. Having healthy skin to start with can optimize the outcomes for any procedure while protecting the skin in the long term. Consider it as protecting your investment.

Dermabrasion, Microdermabrasion, and Skin Peels

Dermabrasion is a more aggressive type of skin peel involving removal of the upper layers of skin through surgical "scraping" of the skin. This treatment is usually reserved for facial wrinkles or scars. Microderm-abrasion is less aggressive, but also uses abrasion to gently "sand" away the uneven outer layer of skin. Microdermabrasion treats sun damage, discoloration, stretch marks, and small scars. Skin peels use a solution to remove the damaged outer layer of skin, helping to improve its texture and tone. These options can refresh the appearance of the skin in both men and women.

Lasering

Lasering is a more aggressive type of treatment. Lasering includes non-ablative, ablative, and micro-ablative.

Non-ablative lasering is a light-based treatment that doesn't really change the structure of the skin but helps with pigment discoloration, sun damage, and vascular lesions. It's basically a light that's attracted to color—it zaps the colored lesions on the skin, not in the skin, and they peel off.

Ablative lasering basically destroys the whole top layer of the skin. A person that has undergone ablative treatment has a waxy, shiny appearance to their skin, mainly due to the destructive nature of the treatment. Ablative lasering was done years ago with aggressive dermabrasion and ablative lasers. It's a treatment that's not done as often anymore because it is so aggressive.

Today, micro-ablative treatment is one of the most common types of laser. These are micro-ablative carbon dioxide lasers that use fractional technology to basically punch microholes in the skin, reducing pore sizes and allowing new skin and growth to occur. The treatment is very similar to aerating a lawn or a golf course, where holes are punched in the grass and new, healthier grass grows. It's the exact same concept with the skin. "Aerating" the skin helps stimulate regrowth of collagen and elastin to tighten the tissue and improve the appearance of skin. Collagen and elastin give skin its elasticity. They change with aging. By inducing heat into the skin at the microlevel, we're trying to get an inflammatory response, which leads to healthy, tightened skin.

The treatment tightens skin and offers mild to moderate improvements in wrinkling. It can be done with the patient awake or asleep; obviously asleep, the treatment can be more aggressive. At my practice, we offer it as a treatment of three sessions so that the patient gets an accumulative effect.

There are also erbium-based and other types of lasers that can be used with the same effect. Erbium lasers tend to be better at discoloration because they don't generate as much heat.

Fillers and Fat Grafting

In terms of the soft-tissue changes, there is a huge market of fillers and fat grafting that freshen your appearance without a long downtime following treatment.

Perhaps the most-publicized type of injectable is Botox, an injection treatment to reduce wrinkles. Botox is tremendously helpful for men, who tend to have very dark, very deep lines and wrinkles.

There are dozens of fillers on the market, but the three main ones are hyaluronic acid, calcium hydroxyapatite based, and autologous fat transfer, which harvests the patient's own fat to be injected into the facial tissues.

Hyaluronic acid is a naturally occurring substance in the body. It's injected into the soft tissue and generally lasts somewhere between nine and fifteen months. It can be injected into folds within the soft tissue, such as the nasal labial or marionette line in the face, and it can be injected into the lips as a plumping agent. On the upside, hyaluronic acid is readily available to a qualified professional and easy to use. The downside is that it is expensive and it lasts a finite amount of time, which varies greatly among people.

Hydroxyapatite is more calcium based, so it is similar to bone structure. It is used in and around areas where we're trying to augment or improve bone structure, such as in the cheekbones or zygomatic arch area (above the jaw), jawline, or chin. Like hyaluronic acid, it's easy for the qualified professional to use, but it's also expensive and has a finite life, usually lasting about twelve months. Plus, most people need a decent volume to make a difference. However, bone fillers tend to last anywhere from one to two years. Again, the goal is to reconstruct or rebuild that deteriorating bone structure in an effort to restore that inverted triangle appearance.

That's really the case with any of these fillers—most people need a decent amount. In other words, they need multiple injections, and that can get expensive quickly. Plus, they last a finite amount of time; they're not permanent.

Autologous fat transfer involves harvesting your own fat, usually around the belly button area, and then injecting it into the face. It can be injected throughout the face: in the cheeks to lift them and give them more fullness, in the forehead to reduce wrinkles, along the nasal labial fold to reduce the line from the edge of the lips to the nose, in the lips to make them plumper, in the tear trough area below the eyes where people get dark circles and sunken appearance—really anywhere on the face in general.

Fat grafting is usually more expensive up front. About 60 percent of the graft survives, and what survives will live with you the rest of your life. Roughly half of patients require two sessions of fat grafting to get the graft to take because the procedure doesn't just inject a large clump of fat. The fat tissue that is being transferred has to be in touch with surrounding vascularized tissue, or tissue that contains blood vessels. If a clump of fat is placed where it is not in touch with the right tissues, then it won't survive. Only the outer parts that are vascularized survive.

Fat grafting is a minimally invasive procedure, so it is done when the patient is awake in a procedure room. The fat is suctioned from the body, strained, and then injected with a very small syringe. Handheld microsuction keeps from damaging the fat during the process.

Recently, fat grafting technology has really improved. Where we used to use larger molecules of fat, we are now performing micro- and nano-fat grafting. The procedure passes the harvested fat through a filtering mechanism, which decreases the particle size, reduces lumpiness and unevenness, and improves the outcome of the procedure.

The fat grafting technique is tailored to the location of the face and the desired outcome. Microfat adds more volume. Autologous fat grafting adds the most volume.

Nano-fat doesn't really increase volume, but it will stimulate new tissue growth and overall health of skin. There is almost no real fat in nanografting; it's actually using stem cells and growth factors to grow new tissue. Skin thins with time. The dermis, or basically the membrane of the skin, becomes thinner, which is what contributes to the less healthy appearance of the skin to the point of the skin becoming translucent. Nano-fat grafting increases the dermal thickness, improving the healthiness and appearance of the skin.

All these methods are aimed at restoring the volume of the face, filling wrinkles at rest, and lifting soft tissue of the face that has dropped due to aging. As I mentioned in the introduction, wrinkles are actually created by shadows, so eliminating them is a matter of managing how they reflect light. Fillers are aimed at trying to soften or lessen those lines to eliminate the deep wrinkles and lines at facial rest that make people look older. (Remember: Botox stops wrinkles that occur when you smile or frown, which is called facial animation. Fillers, on the other hand, fill lines you have when your face is at rest without expression.)

Over time, however, fillers may not be adequate, and that's when we get into minimally invasive and all-out invasive surgery. These range from the incision of skin and tightening of skin to full-on neck and face lifts, where we try to resuspend and replace those structures to where they originally were. Again, the goal is to restore that inverted triangle.

Noninvasive or Minimally Invasive Surgery

Some simple surgery options can be done very quickly and with minimal downtime and recovery. These work well for women and men, and include blepharoplasty or eyelid surgery that can correct sagging and drooping eyelids that come with aging and puffiness under the eyes, which can make a person look very tired or even angry.

One of these options is energy-assisted liposuction using deoxycholic acid, which is a man-made form of a fat-absorbing substance in your body; deoxycholic acid destroys fat cells wherever it is injected. Energy-assisted liposuction is a great option for tightening the jowl, which can age the face in men and women as it gets heavier over time. This procedure, sometimes known as double-chin surgery or a mini–neck lift, results in tighter skin on the neck and a more defined chin. Deoxycholic acid works well for reducing male breast tissue, something we're seeing more often at my practice. The treatment is done through a few small incisions, making it less traumatic than treatments of the past. The patient can then wear compression under his shirt and return to work within a few days.

Body contouring using a procedure known as cryolipolysis, or CoolSculpting, involves "freezing away" fat. This is something that men and women choose for the "love handles" that develop as metabolism slows with aging and fat deposition increases around the midsection.

These are some of the options for helping men age more subtly, and helping women maintain or more aggressively turn back the clock—especially those in public-facing roles, such as sales or public relations. In fact, we're seeing women in their twenties and thirties coming in for Botox and skin-care treatments because they are more aware of how they appear and how that impacts their careers.

The key with any of these treatments is to match it to the patient's needs and wants. When we have a patient come in who's not happy with how they look, whose exterior doesn't match their interior, then we can review their situation and determine a treatment that will begin to turn back the clock. For those who have already been through a treatment by another provider and are unhappy with their results, we often find that it's because the procedure really was not the right one for their situation.

With any procedure, communication between the surgeon and the patient is key; it plays a crucial role in a successful cosmetic plastic surgery experience.

"NOTHING MAKES
A WOMAN MORE
BEAUTIFUL THAN
THE BELIEF THAT
SHE IS BEAUTIFUL."

—SOPHIA LOREN

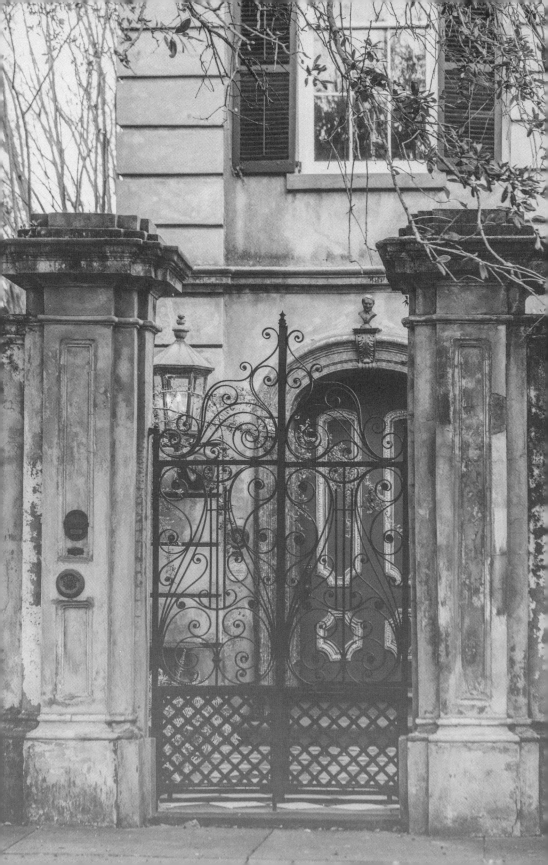

CHAPTER 4

"How Can I Live with This?"

IS THIS FLAW KEEPING ME FROM BEING "BEAUTIFUL"?

Sharon came to see me asking for help with a scar from an abdominoplasty, commonly known as a tummy tuck. She had undergone the procedure some months prior, and the results were actually great: her abdomen was flat, her clothes fit her well, and her posture had even improved since she was no longer carrying all the weight around her midsection.

Prior to the procedure, we had discussed in depth what she could reasonably expect. There would be scarring, I explained, because making an incision in human skin causes a scar. That is unavoidable. Plastic surgery involves taking away skin or stretching and moving skin, and that means trading your current physical condition for a scar. Over time, the appearance of the scar will improve, but it will likely always be there, or at least take a very long time to disappear completely. Depending on the condition of the scar, there are procedures that we may be able to perform down the road—after nine to twelve months—to improve the appearance of the scar.

When Sharon showed me the scar, it was about as would be expected for the procedure she had undergone. Although visible, it was not what many would consider to be a "horrible" scar. So it took me a bit of question-and-answer to understand her real concerns.

She hesitated to explain her concerns further. Finally, she blurted out that the scar was "wrecking her marriage." "My husband doesn't want to be with me anymore because of that scar," she said.

What Sharon was dealing with clearly went deeper than the scar on her abdomen. Sharon was dealing with that twofold definition of beauty. While so many people see beauty as purely an outward, physical attribute, there is also that unseen beauty, that belief in a person's own self-worth. That is a beauty that lies within. It is something no one else can give you, and no one else can determine for you. You cannot improve physical attributes enough to make anyone see something inside you that does not transcend your physical features or limitations.

As discussed earlier, when it comes to using cosmetic plastic surgery to achieve beauty, happy patients are those who have a realistic understanding of the end goals of their procedures. What are we trying to achieve? Larger breasts? A smaller nose? Less sag under the chin?

> When it comes to using cosmetic plastic surgery to achieve beauty, happy patients are those who have a realistic understanding of the end goals of their procedures.

Whatever the objective, whatever the expectation, it must be realistic. That's the responsibility of the plastic surgeon: to determine whether the patient goals are achievable and safe.

Unfortunately, patients seeking plastic surgery sometimes do so because they are intent on "fixing" what they perceive to be a physical "flaw" that is often so small it is barely visible to others—minor wrinkles and small scars are common. Sometimes the "flaw" is something others rarely see, since it is usually concealed by clothing. Often, it is something others do not view as a "flaw" at all. I am constantly amazed at how people see themselves compared to what other people see. That is probably the single biggest source of dissatisfaction or unhappiness—but it's an altered perception and one that can ultimately affect the outcome. Many people are overly critical of their own images, and they believe what they think is what others are thinking as well—and that's usually not the case. Most of the time, people don't criticize others; they just don't make the effort to be critical. People are usually so wrapped up in their own lives they just don't have the time, or interest, to focus on someone else. So they're certainly not going to notice something like a small wrinkle.

With the various procedures available through cosmetic plastic surgery, we can usually improve an area of a person's physical appearance that may be keeping them up at night. Whether it is a wrinkle, a small blemish, or a minor deformity, chances are we have a procedure that can improve whatever is felt to be a physical imperfection. But when a small imperfection is not the root of the problem, chances are the patient will not be happy, no matter what procedure we perform.

I'm not talking about a clearly noticeable disfiguration. Some people spend all, or a good portion, of their lives dealing with a prominent physical deformity. Some people are born with a disfigurement, while others end up with one following an accident or disease. When a person's physical appearance causes a genuine stigma, there certainly may be options for improvement, pain relief, and ideally, help with achieving a more active and social life.

It's interesting, though, that people with altered or even grossly deformed physical appearances often seem to be more comfortable with who they are. Their families, friends, and spouses still see them as beautiful. When they seek plastic surgery, often it's for functional improvement: they want to improve their quality of life. The aesthetics are often a secondary concern.

However, there is obviously something misaligned in someone who feels just as strongly about a small wrinkle or blemish as someone who, for instance, is suffering from the scars of third-degree burns. People who are overly concerned with small blemishes tend to feel that the world is against them, that nothing in their life is ever "right." For someone who is letting a small physical feature impact their life in a negative way, we can perform procedures to help improve that physical feature, but chances are great that they are still going to feel the same about themselves after recovery, or they will find another problem, something else about their body that they deem unacceptable. Ultimately, if something bothers a patient, I don't believe it is my responsibility as the surgeon to tell the patient what they should or should not have done, but I believe I have a responsibility to address three issues:

1. Can I see the problem, and do I understand their concern?

2. Is there a viable option to address the problem that they see?

3. Is the treatment option safe and in the best interest of the patient?

The truth is that people usually see themselves quite differently from the way everyone else sees them. Some may see the tiniest line on their face and claim it's a flaw they can't live with; it may be a line so small the surgeon has to squint to see it. When a patient is hypercritical, I have concerns. There is no guarantee anything I do will make them better, and in fact, anything I do may be perceived by the patient as making the blemish worse. Patient perception is key.

Some of that self-misperception can be a real challenge to address. Gloria, for instance, came to see me, wanting a tummy tuck after losing ninety pounds but plateauing in her weight loss. She felt that a tummy tuck would take her to the next level in her journey to better health. Unfortunately, even after that significant and commendable weight loss, Gloria still weighed 290 pounds. As she was five feet six inches tall, that was still too much weight for her frame. Although she was very happy with her current weight, and I was very happy for her progress, she was still considered to be morbidly obese, and that had to factor into my consideration of whether plastic surgery was the best option for her. At the age of thirty, except for her weight, she could have been considered healthy enough to heal relatively well since she did not smoke or have high blood pressure, high cholesterol, diabetes, or other significant health issues.

In the end, there was really no way to meet her expectations. That's because there are two types of belly fat: visceral and subcutaneous. Visceral fat, also known as intra-abdominal fat, is located inside the abdominal cavity, where it wraps around your body's organs. Unfortunately, no surgery can remove visceral fat. The only way to lose it is by losing weight through better nutrition and exercise. Subcutaneous fat, on the other hand, is outside the abdominal wall and just underneath the skin. Subcutaneous fat can be removed by cosmetic plastic surgery. Gloria's body still had too much visceral fat. It would have been physically impossible for a tummy tuck to give her the flat belly she envisioned. In addition, her risk for complications from the procedure far outweighed the potential benefits.

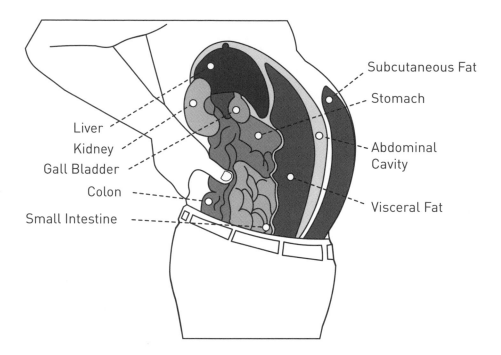

Liver
Kidney
Gall Bladder
Colon
Small Intestine

Subcutaneous Fat
Stomach
Abdominal
Cavity
Visceral Fat

Misaligned self-images and misaligned emotions are reasons for my being very cautious when working with teens on their still-changing bodies. Depending on their age, teenagers are usually still growing and changing, not only physically but also mentally and emotionally. For instance, it's difficult to justify plastic surgery on a fourteen-year-old girl who doesn't like her nose or whose breasts have not yet developed.

Yet it's not entirely uncommon for teens that young to seriously consider cosmetic plastic surgery. Why? Technology is obviously changing rapidly and, with it, dramatically evolving the way we live. One area, of course, is social media, and the groups that may be most impacted are children and teens. As a cosmetic plastic surgeon, I'm in a unique position to really see the impact that social media is making on young people—and every year it seems to be impacting more people at a younger age.

As I mentioned in chapter 1, social media is immersing children and teens in a world that they may not be mature enough to understand. We've all heard stories about youth being bullied on social media because of their appearances, whether that's due to physical features or the clothes they wear.

Where cosmetic plastic surgery becomes a part of the picture is when teens idolize people whom they see in social media. The problem is that the fame those social media "stars" enjoy is based on endorsing products or a certain look. As a result, they are constantly changing their appearance as a way of adhering to their obligation to that online presence. Teens are seeing how people on social media *ooh* and *ah* over someone because of their sculpted bum or fuller lips, and they're seeing how people use cosmetic plastic surgery—fillers, Botox, and other procedures—to change their looks or feel better about themselves. It's all enforcing the message in already-bullied children and teens that they're not good enough if they don't look a certain way, perhaps impacting a youth's self-esteem and even leading to more bullying.

Again, the problem is that they want to be like those people they see on social media, but they don't understand that a lot of what they're seeing is not necessarily real. They're idolizing supermodels and social media superstars without realizing that images online are often manipulated using Photoshop or filters. They don't understand that people with very high-profile images that rely on looks know how to look good when they are in public. They know how best to move and pose; they know how the light makes them look and how to accommodate for it. Nobody wakes up in the morning and crawls out of bed looking like a superstar. But youth who don't have a grasp of that reality think that they're the ones with the issue; that places additional pressure and stress on them and can make them more insecure than they already are at a time when they should be enjoying life and not worrying about being a little gawky. They're at an age when their bodies and minds are still developing, but they are hyperfocused on what is still essentially a work in progress. They don't comprehend that those images they're seeing are designed to sell an image, to be clickbait based on shock value—the people they are viewing are supported by the number of followers they get online. It's a cycle—they change their looks, dramatize what they're doing, get more followers, get more clicks, get more advertisers interested because of those followers, and ultimately make more money. These celebrities have millions of followers because they're portraying something that's attractive to the masses. But that something may not be real, and it may not be true.

Why is all this happening? Social media has become the battle-field where people fight to be noticed. They gauge their self-worth and popularity on how many followers they have or likes they get from a post. They see influencers and celebrities portraying a certain type of a look or lifestyle and try to mimic that in the hopes of being popular. Unfortunately, social media is the perfect avenue for fake and disingenuous information, which a younger person may not notice or realize. The lack of age guidelines on social media has allowed young people to be exposed to many things on social media they may not fully understand or may not be mature enough to understand yet. Filters, Photoshop, and fake posts now allow any user to become someone they are not in an effort to impress those around them. They begin to chase a fantasy, and some turn to cosmetic plastic surgery for help.

I have performed cosmetic procedures on teens when I believed there was a deficit or a defect that could be improved. But in those cases, it comes down to the maturity of the patient. They seemed to very clearly understand what they were having done and why and to the best of their ability, the risks and benefits of it. Anyone under age eighteen is a minor, and that means a parent or guardian has to approve the procedure, so their involvement is crucial. The adult must be present in the consult because they know their child better than I can get to know them in a consult.

When a patient is a minor, one factor I look for is whether there is any indication that the parent desires their teen to have the procedure more so than the patient. I've had consults where the parent does all the talking, and in those situations, I make sure to specifically ask the teen: "Why are you here? What do you want?" When I ask them, I want to hear them answer, not the parent. If a teen can't seem to answer my questions—maybe because they are too shy or timid—then I try to talk with them to help them feel a little more comfortable with the situation. But at some point, if they just can't verbalize what they want and why, then they probably should not have the procedure done because there are just too many risks involved. For instance, they could end up with a scar in an area of their body that they already didn't like. As you'll read in the chapters ahead, the fact that there are no guarantees in cosmetic plastic surgery is a concept that even adults have trouble grasping, so it usually takes a very mature teen to rationalize having a procedure done, considering all the complications that can occur.

Again, young bodies are still developing, so there are certain areas of the body and certain procedures that should not be done on younger folks because they're still growing and maturing. In most cases, I prefer to wait until someone is of legal age to voice their desires and to consent to the procedure itself. Even then, many young people really don't have the capacity to fully understand what they're getting into.

That said, most of the time, when a teen and parent come in for a consult, it's about something that has been bothering them both for some time. In fact, that's the reason one of the first questions I typically ask is "How long has this been bothering you?" If they answer, "Since last week," then that's a red flag. But if they tell me they've been talking about it for six months, a year, or "for as long as I can remember," then I feel there is a level of commitment that warrants further discussion.

Another part of what I look for in the consult is whether there is an expectation of immediate gratification—they think they're going to have the procedure on Monday and wake up Tuesday looking exactly as they envision. Especially when someone's expectations are set by social media, there is often that sense of immediacy—all that clicking makes it seem like change happens in an instant. What's not understood is that, even though it seems like daily updates on favorite celebrities are available, there can be huge gaps of time between pictures that are posted. Photos may be posted days apart, but the real time lapse may be several months. That celebrity's new look may not have been a linear journey; they may have had additional procedures done to revise their initial outcomes.

So how does a parent talk to a teen about plastic surgery when maybe they are considering having something done themselves? It really depends on family culture and dynamics, as well as perhaps even which part of the country you may live in. For instance, there is a much different view of looks where I practice in the conservative South compared to a city like Miami, New York, or Los Angeles. Where such discussions often occur is when genetics are involved—a young adult may want to have something done if, at an early age, they look in the mirror and they start to see a family trait that they know will soon make them look older than their age. In some instances, parents may think it doesn't matter since they never addressed the issue, but to the next generation, it may really matter.

Seeing a familiar aging feature in the face can especially be an issue if it involves someone's career. That's why I really want to know what's important to the person when they come in for a consult. I performed energy-assisted liposuction and an upper eyelid procedure on a nineteen-year-old model from New York. She may have weighed 115 pounds at the time but was beginning to develop a bit of fat under her chin, and her eyes were beginning to look heavy and hooded. In Charleston, where I practice, there are few careers that would have someone thinking twice about that little bit of extra chin and a difference in their eyes at age nineteen, although later in adulthood, they certainly consider having these procedures done.

Again, what will make you happy? Why are you considering a procedure, and what is your end goal? If I ask those questions and the answers are pulled up on a smartphone—to look like a picture of a filtered Instagram star—that's not a good sign. If they want Kylie Jenner's lips or Kim Kardashian's bum, then there's a problem; there are five billion people in the world, and to believe that a small procedure is going to make you look like someone else and that's going to make you happy is a concern. If, however, they don't like the way their nose looks in pictures and they actually do have an unattractive bump, then I think that's a reasonable request. It's something factual and fixable, it's been bothering them for some time, and fixing it would make them happy.

If someone is over age eighteen and can consent for themselves, that's a different argument, unless they need the parents financially. Then the parents are obviously enabling them, and that's when the discussion then has to look at the parents' motives. Is there really a valid reason, or is it just because their child wants to look like their favorite celebrity? Remember: What's in style today won't be in style twenty years from today, and even celebrities know that.

However, there are conditions in teens that can be addressed more aggressively with plastic surgery. These include breast development issues such as gynecomastia in boys or macromastia in girls. Gynecomastia is abnormal swelling of breast tissue caused by a hormonal imbalance. Macromastia is one form of breast hypertrophy, or excessive enlargement of the breasts. Both of these conditions can affect teens' development emotionally and psychologically because to them and to their peers, these conditions are sometimes considered to be physical deformities. Both conditions can keep teens from participating in school activities, such as sports. And for girls, macromastia can even lead to physical issues such as neck and back pain.

Plastic surgery can also address other teen issues such as scars caused by animal bites or trauma, since scars can affect their socialization and ultimately have an impact on a teen's emotional development.

Constricted breast, a congenital breast deformity in which only one breast develops normally and creates significant asymmetry, is another issue that can be resolved with plastic surgery. Constricted breast, typically, becomes an issue just beyond the teen years, when a young woman is entering college, starting in the workforce, or planning to get married.

The good news is that teens' expectations often seem more aligned with the realities of plastic surgery. They are more likely to take everything in stride and be happy with their results, unless other kids make fun of them. As bullying and body shaming become more prevalent in the mainstream media, I believe plastic surgery, in the right setting, can be used to educate and hopefully help through education and information, not necessarily by doing procedures on adolescents who are not ready mentally or physically for that type of dramatic and permanent change.

As a parent of four daughters and also a plastic surgeon, I find the discussion about appearance and perception fascinating. I think letting teens be open with their questions and opinions regarding both social media and physical appearance is important. If they don't feel they can be open with you as their parent, then they will find another avenue for information and advice, and it most likely won't be a source that is best for them. Pretending that social media and body image are not related and greatly impacting your child nearly all the time is shortsighted at best.

I have had children and adolescents brought in by their families to discuss such things as ear surgery for prominent ears or surgery for gynecomastia (male breast development). In some cases, surgery is a viable option; however, in others, I have used the consultation as an opportunity to tell the patient they don't need surgery and that they are normal. Oftentimes, hearing this from a stranger, and to some degree a plastic surgeon, not their family, has been helpful. Children are so impressionable and sensitive to the opinions of their peers; I want to do whatever I can to help them feel better in their own skin. I hate hearing how a child is impacted by being teased or bullied regarding appearance; I guess I know from seeing them as a patient how deeply it hurts them, and to hear what often happens at school is heartbreaking.

Ironically, using a plastic surgeon to help reassure a child that they are normal and that they don't need anything done, despite kids at school thinking otherwise, is a great teaching opportunity.

Adults, on the other hand, often have more trouble aligning their expectations, especially those who have trouble coming to grips with the reality of their life situations. Women and men going through midlife crises and worried about the first signs of wrinkles may have unreasonable expectations about what plastic surgery can do for them.

Unrealistic expectations in midlife may stem from some of the same issues someone has at an earlier age: poor body image, a relationship falling apart, or overwhelming stresses that alter state of mind. And just like a developing teen, whose emotions are sometimes in upheaval, an adult reaching middle age and dealing with declining hormones may have a constantly changing outlook on life.

As I mentioned in chapter 2, genetics certainly can play a role in plastic surgery outcomes and can also play a role in how a person ages—both good and bad. Again, at some point in life, many people see a parent when they look in the mirror. Genetics can determine similarities in how the face, skin, and body ages. Everyone has the potential to age as other members of their family do. Ethnicity can also be a determining factor. For instance, people from the Mediterranean region tend to have "thicker," oilier skin, which can be more hydrating and appear healthier longer. While that may mean dealing with more acne and breakouts in childhood, it can also mean having fewer wrinkles in old age.

Whatever the body type or reason for pursuing plastic surgery, it is crucial to understand that there is a difference between seeing or thinking something is beautiful and truly feeling beauty. The feeling of beauty comes from a combination of improving a perceived physical flaw while cultivating your own true inner beauty. Cosmetic plastic surgery can free a person from the grip of insecurity that may arise from a physical flaw the patient has held on to and consequently allow their inner self to emerge. It is crucial to understand before undergoing any procedure that thinking, seeing, and feeling beautiful is about what is on the inside. Sometimes surgery can just help you remove barriers that are preventing your best self from coming forward.

A positive outlook can significantly affect healing and the ultimate outcome of any procedure. I can't emphasize that enough. I've seen time and time again how a patient's mental and emotional state going into surgery has had a dramatic effect on how fast and well they recover and heal from the procedure. People who have less emotional scarring tend to have smoother recoveries and better outcomes. While I can't say from a medical standpoint that a patient can will, or think, himself or herself into being healed or having a successful surgery, I do believe patients with better outlooks and more motivation tend to recover quicker and have better outcomes.

In other words, people who are organized, motivated, and healthier, or are even overachievers in other areas of life, tend to breeze through the process. They tend to eat better and exercise more. They tend to be more active after surgery. They seem to have a more realistic view of the outcomes to be expected and are likely to listen intently during the consultation, read through the literature, and follow post-operative directions. They take more responsibility for their healing.

Conversely, for people who are unorganized and unhealthy, and who tend to blame the world for their problems, the surgery itself can become a source of lament. Depressed, angry people may not eat or exercise as well. They may almost expect something to go wrong. Instead of getting up and being active after surgery, they may lie around and stress eat, waiting for the first hint of a perceived "imperfection," which then may set them on a perceived course of failure: "Here we go again. Everything always goes wrong for me." That mentality can greatly slow the healing process and overall makes patients unhappy. People with that kind of mindset tend to give the consultation, literature, and postoperative recovery instructions lip service and then show up two weeks after a procedure complaining that it wasn't what they expected.

The truth is that surgery doesn't have the ability to rationalize. It doesn't choose who it's going to be successful for and who it's going to fail. Surgery is a physical process in which healing proceeds at different rates depending on multiple factors that vary with each patient. Many of those factors are out of the control of both the surgeon and the patient.

Similarly, body fat doesn't have the power to choose where it resides in the body. Adults have a fixed number of fat cells. Liposuction removes fat cells. Performing liposuction in one area removes some of the cells from that area. Contrary to what many people believe, having liposuction in one area of the body doesn't mean fat will move around to other areas; fat's not that smart. There's a physiological reason why fat cells show or don't: they get bigger or smaller based on the number of calories a person consumes. It's like a checking account. If you write a lot of checks but don't deposit any money into your account, the funds in your account will shrink. Your account will be smaller at the end of the day, but you'll still have the account. Put some money into the account, and it will grow. The same concept applies to fat. If you burn more calories than you take in, your fat cells will shrink and appear smaller. But if you take in a lot of calories, your fat cells will grow larger.

When it comes to elective surgery, patients must remember that it's a choice, one that they must accept responsibility for and be prepared to see through to its completion.

I liken plastic surgery and the responsibility involved to bariatric surgery. After a gastric bypass, patients who follow the process will lose a lot of weight, crazy fast. But it is possible to eat around a bypass. Unfortunately, people who do that usually gain back all the weight they lost and then some. Gastric bypass is a good example of how surgery can only do so much. Gastric bypass patients must undergo extensive psychological analysis prior to the surgery, and they must have a strong support network. Even with those components in the process, it's up to the patients to do their part in ensuring the surgery succeeds.

Simply put, plastic surgery will not always fix an ailing self-image, it won't fix relationships, it won't change what other people think of you, and on its own, it won't turn your life completely around. If someone finds fault with you, causing you to consider cosmetic plastic surgery, consider whether that procedure will actually change that person's view of you. More importantly, will that procedure make you happy? When a minor imperfection seems to be negatively impacting your life and causing you great distress, it may be time to not only pause and look for the real beauty in you, but also see if the problem can be addressed in a safe and efficient way that allows you to be happy with yourself inside and out.

> When it comes to elective surgery, patients must remember that it's a choice, one that they must accept responsibility for and be prepared to see through to its completion.

People who are dissatisfied are often motivated to take action. When that dissatisfaction leads to unrealistic expectations of cosmetic plastic surgery outcomes, I sometimes have to share with patients that they may not be the best candidate for a procedure. That is one of the toughest parts of being a plastic surgeon. But when dissatisfaction brings me people in search of options for realistically improving their appearance, I am extremely happy to help them try to achieve their objectives.

"ONE OF THE MOST COURAGEOUS DECISIONS YOU'LL EVER MAKE IS TO FINALLY LET GO OF WHAT IS HURTING YOUR HEART AND SOUL."

—BRIGITTE NICOLE

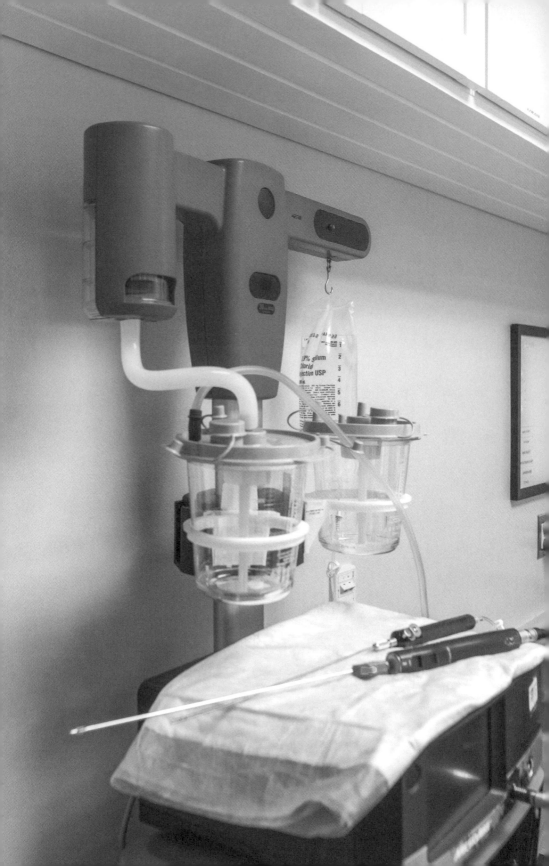

CHAPTER 5

"You're the One Who Wanted to Do This"

HOW DO I PREPARE MY FAMILY FOR THIS JOURNEY WITH ME?

W hen it comes to cosmetic plastic surgery, it's important that it's not being done to impress anyone else—friends, family, partners, or anyone else. It's got to be for you—and only you. Yet during the postoperative healing process, it really takes the support of others, especially family.

In fact, family members play an important role in cosmetic plastic surgery both pre- and postoperatively. In addition to the physical aspects of healing, family members must understand that patients are vulnerable and emotionally drained after surgery. Their bodies are in a tough place due to the stress of surgery and the effects of postoperative care and medications. But they are also experiencing a roller coaster of emotions, including regret, uncertainty, and the overwhelming fear of having made a mistake. Even the strongest, most stable person can be tremendously rattled by the surgical experience.

That's why the support of family members and loved ones is crucial. Yet it can be a real challenge to get family on board for several reasons.

For starters, family members may not agree with your desire to have something done in the first place. In chapter 8, I talk about how family members often have trouble understanding why their beloved wants to have something done when "they're already perfect."

But if you're the one considering cosmetic plastic surgery, think about it as you would when buying yourself a car. You're not going to choose it based on someone else's favorite color or other features; you're going to buy it to your own liking, to your own specific situation. What one person likes or wants or needs may not fit someone else. And that's OK—it's OK to want something that is different than what others want.

Therein is the challenge: you're not doing this for your family, so getting their buy-in—and their support—is no small task. Family and loved ones are often hesitant; they are scared of the unknown and worried about you as a patient. After all, any type of surgery is both physically and mentally taxing. And it can be tough for family members to understand when it is not as much about physical health as it is about mental outlook. Preparing for cosmetic plastic surgery— and even through recovery—is both an emotional and physical experience. That's why a positive outlook for both patient and family members is so important.

In fact, considering all there is to know and do before and after the surgery, the whole process can be difficult for patients, and overwhelming for family members—most of whom are not medical people. Although they may want to help, they're worried about the patient; they're worried that they're going to do something wrong. There can be a lot of family members who often have the mindset that "We already loved you as you were" or "You're the one who wanted to do this."

The mental and emotional state of patient and family members has a dramatic effect on healing and recovery, and the process as a whole. Better outcomes tend to be the results when there is less emotional scarring from the start. People who have a healthy outlook and a strong support system seem to have more realistic expectations and are happier with their results than people who tend to blame the world for their problems and have family members who are not there for them mentally or emotionally.

> Preparing for cosmetic plastic surgery—and even through recovery—is both an emotional and physical experience. That's why a positive outlook for both patient and family members is so important.

That's why it's so important at the very beginning to know that you're not doing it for somebody else. It's about you and the quality of life you envision after the procedure. Yes, it's elective surgery. And yes, it's only for you. But it's important to get family on board early on. Patients are already mentally in a tough spot afterward because they're not feeling great; they obviously don't look great yet, and because of the way they feel, they may even be questioning their motives themselves. Then to have others saying, "Well, you did this to yourself" does not help in their healing process.

Stress and anxiety impact healing by causing vasoconstriction, or restricted blood flow, and by releasing catecholamines such as cortisol, the stress hormone, in the bloodstream. That can significantly impede the body's ability to heal in a timely manner. Whether that stress is "self-induced"—in other words, the patient is a naturally anxious person—or it's coming from external factors, such as stress in their personal or professional life, it can impact how a cosmetic plastic surgery incision heals.

So in addition to physical preparation and proper nutrition, addressing emotional concerns and having a caring environment postsurgery are all crucial to healing.

An integral part of pre- and postoperative preparation is counseling—for the patient and family members. While it's important for anyone in an elevated emotional state, it's especially important for patients who have high levels of anxiety or bipolar disorder because surgery can sometimes trigger an episode. People with very high anxiety don't typically handle any form of setback very well, even perceived setbacks. When it comes to cosmetic plastic surgery, the mentality that "This always happens to me" or "I have the worst luck" or "This isn't going to work" is always very difficult because the expected change that surgery will bring about takes time. Improvements aren't seen in hours or days following surgery; they're gradual, occurring over weeks and months (or even a year, for scarring). So it's very important to address the psychological tie to immediacy.

Similarly, people who are chronic worriers and have anxiety as a baseline often have family interactions that are already a little stressed.

In spite of a stigma about counseling, in my practice, we have a counselor available to talk with patients to help with anxiety and stress levels, and we are one of the very few plastic surgery offices across the United States to add a counselor to our staff. I believe this support mechanism is invaluable to both the patient and the patient's family, before and after surgery. Even when a patient is emotionally stable and has good family support, we still recommend establishing a relationship or a line of communication with the counselor prior to the procedure. That way, the relationship is already in place in case it's needed later. Since surgery is such a focused stress event, it's good to know there is someone to turn to should you ultimately need them.

Once you have addressed the emotional side of the equation, then it's time to get with the surgeon and have a dialogue about the actual procedure and postsurgery. When meeting with the surgeon, it's always good to have some family members in attendance so that everyone better understands the risks, the benefits, the likely outcomes. It's best for everyone to hear firsthand what might be an imperfect scenario, and what likely is to happen.

When sitting down with the surgeon, look for them to provide information on what to expect after the procedure, including care considerations and a timeline. I share more about both of these later in this chapter.

Next are the physical preparations. Prior to surgery, obviously, it's important to get medical clearance. That depends on your situation and may involve visiting your primary care doctor to have labs done and potentially undergo an EKG or other types of tests. Many cosmetic plastic surgeries are performed in the office, but they are done with IV sedation. It's not what is often envisioned as surgery, with a hospital stay, endotracheal tubes and intubation, and being paralyzed. It's a much different process.

The medications are basically the same used in colonoscopies or dental office procedures, so it's a much gentler experience than undergoing anesthesia during major surgery in a hospital. There is no real "hangover" effect, and most people say it's the best rest they've had in a long time.

Typically, in advance of surgery, when patients sign the consent form, we issue the prescription that the patient will need postsurgery. That way they can have it filled and ready to go when they get home after the procedure. As part of preparations for your procedure, be sure to discuss in detail with your surgeon and anesthesiologist the following concerns:

- any medications that you take, including naturopathic or home remedies

- any allergic reactions you've had with medications

- any previous experience with anesthesia, including any post-procedure nausea or extreme grogginess

It's crucial to be very open with your provider about the types of medications that you take so that you can be properly informed on what can continue to be taken, what should be stopped in advance, and when you can begin taking your medications after the procedure. Over-the-counter pain medications like Motrin or Tylenol can be adjusted on an individual basis, but it's a good idea to let your primary care doctors or other specialists know that you're undergoing a procedure in order to get their recommendations for any medications that they've prescribed. That way the cosmetic plastic surgeon can work with your other physicians to determine what's best for you postprocedure.

For example, while blood thinners can cause a higher risk of bleeding, I don't always stop them before a procedure. Why? I'd rather have to deal with a hematoma, or a little extra bleeding, than have someone develop a blood clot or have a stroke because they stopped their blood thinner.

The key message is transparency. It's important for patients to be completely open about what they ingest because even over-the-counter supplements like fish oil can sometimes interact with anesthesia. While it can sometimes be embarrassing for a patient to talk about a smoking, alcohol, or drug habit, it's vitally important for physicians, surgeons, and anesthesia providers to know about these because of the complications they can cause. I would rather know if someone has a few drinks daily because asking them to stop can cause withdrawals, which can unnecessarily complicate recovery. Another problem is that too often patients take a narcotic sedative the night before a procedure to calm their nerves and fail to inform the surgeon or anesthesiologist because they think it's no big deal. But those can compound the effects of the anesthesia and make it more difficult to arouse someone after a procedure. There are many workarounds we can employ as long as we know what we're dealing with, and that means being completely open and honest with your surgeon before a procedure.

> The key message is transparency. It's important for patients to be completely open about what they ingest.

Beyond the medical components, nutrition is one factor to consider before and after surgery. We recommend increasing protein intake before surgery. We don't want patients trying to lose weight two weeks before surgery and having their body in starvation mode. Before surgery, we also recommend that patients consume 1.5 grams of protein per kilogram of body weight through whatever source works best for them, whether that's a steak or a smoothie. We also want patients to stay hydrated, whether through water or a drink such as Pedialyte or Gatorade, which contains electrolytes.

In addition to presurgery protein, there are dietary recommendations postsurgery. People generally are not hungry after surgery. They lose their appetite for a few weeks, and that's OK. But they still need to get protein to promote healing. Again, the protein can be through a steak meal, if a patient has the appetite, or it can be through other dietary measures such as bars or powders used to make smoothies. We recommend eating a low-pH diet of lean meats, vegetables, and fruits and avoid eating high-fat, high-sugar, processed foods.

Hydration is also crucial postsurgery, and if a patient is someone who already finds it difficult to drink enough water in a day's time, then, again, Pedialyte or Gatorade are good options.

When it comes to alcohol, there are two main concerns postsurgery: we don't want patients mixing alcohol with certain medications, and we don't want them drinking to the point of becoming unstable. After all it's taken to arrive at that point in their journey, we don't want them falling and potentially injuring themselves or the area where they've had a procedure.

Physical activity prior to the procedure is also important because no matter how good your health or physical condition, you're going to get set back by the surgery. In fact, people who are especially active can be affected by inactivity following surgery. More than just the physical aspect, being inactive makes them mentally miserable, and that worsens the healing process. That's one of the top things I hear from patients postsurgery—they're very surprised at how much a cosmetic plastic surgery procedure sets them back physically. In fact, a friend of mine who is an orthopedic surgeon and just recently retired even told me how amazed he was following his hip replacement—a procedure he had performed on patients for thirty years. He's in great shape and works out every day, but he was just astonished at how much the surgery set him back.

Whatever the regimen of walking, exercising, or regular movement is ahead of surgery, find out from the surgeon a timeline of when you can get back on schedule afterward. How strenuously can you move, in what timeframe? Be honest with yourself and others about what it's going to take to heal. Patients often tell us, "I'm a quick healer," but are still surprised at how long it really takes to recover.

More and more I believe physical preparation prior to surgery is crucial to a quick and successful recovery, so much so that when opening new offices now, I have a gym attached to the office and either run the gym through our practice or partner with a third-party gym owner. Having preselected trainers familiar with plastic surgery available to help patients prepare for surgery physically through nutrition and exercise, as well as having them monitor and guide their return to physical activity, is crucial. I think it is safer for the patient and leads to better outcomes.

It's also important for healing to have the family and home prepared for potential physical needs and even some level of incapacity postsurgery. Postsurgery, patients are often draining blood or other body fluid, and it can be a bit of a mess for everyone involved. We recommend that patients cover car seats and furniture at home with bed pads or even shower curtains to prepare for the drainage. Other considerations include the following:

- **Daily meals.** How will meals be prepared, served, and eaten postsurgery? And who's going to clean up afterward?

- **Daily chores.** What other daily activities will you need help with?

- **Pets.** If you have pets, who's going to care for them? Who's going to feed and water them or take care of other needs that they have? There won't be any walking the dog or even letting them jump on you for at least a few days. Will you be able to keep them in the home while you heal, or is there a concern about them being underfoot?

- **The kids.** This one is pretty obvious, and most people have this one covered. But don't forget about things like shuttling the kids to and from school or activities, making sure they get their meals and sleep, and even that they have clean clothes to wear—just doing laundry may be a challenge for a few days, yet too often, moms think they are superwomen who can wake up the next day without a hitch in their schedule. But the healing and recovery process is much easier and less stressful for everyone involved if you have a plan—and help lined up—in advance.

- **Return-to-work schedule.** Have in advance a realistic time expectation of when you'll be able to get back to normal and return to work.

On the day of surgery, the patient and caregiver should receive postoperative instructions. If the instructions are unclear, then ask for clarity before leaving the office. It's crucial to have a precise understanding of the instructions, especially the medication regimen, so that there's no risk of confusion about what to take when, and what can be taken together. Also ensure you have a point of contact—during and after business hours—for any questions. I even recommend having the caregiver audio- and/or video-record discharge instructions from the nurse prior to being discharged; that way they can refer back to them at home if they are confused or uncertain. It can be a lot of information to take in and somewhat overwhelming.

For the first twenty-four hours following surgery with anesthesia, we want the patient to be accompanied by someone at all times.

Here are some other important postoperative care considerations, some of which may involve family members:

- **Expect a low-grade fever.** Surgical procedures are often followed by a low-grade fever. This may be caused by inflammation or may be a residual of the anesthesia administered prior to surgery, which can affect the lungs' ability to absorb oxygen. Patients should reach out to the plastic surgeon who performed their procedure if they have a fever in excess of 101.5 degrees Fahrenheit for twenty-four hours or more. Often, there is no cause for alarm, but it is best to get checked to ensure everything is healing as it should and no challenges are developing.

- **In general, use ice, not heat, for swelling.** Heating pads or hot compresses should be avoided until the plastic surgeon gives the "all clear" to use them. An ice pack applied to the area for short intervals can help reduce the inflammation, but care should be taken when using ice packs. Since the area is numb following surgery, it can be difficult to feel the cold, and too much cold applied too close to the skin can actually cause injury. The skin should be protected from the ice pack by a towel or other material, and the ice pack should be applied for only a limited amount of time to avoid damage to the procedure site.

  Occasionally, warm compresses are used to help incision lines, especially areas that may have a suture abscess or mild cellulitis (bacterial skin infection). Heat causes dilatation of the blood vessels and increased blood flow to wound edges.

- **Take a warm shower.** Showering after surgery can make you feel better. We allow you to shower twenty-four to seventy-two hours following surgery. Baths are not allowed, and pool and ocean water must be avoided, initially, and based on recovery adjusted for each patient. The ideal setup is one that includes a removable shower head that you can use to spray your body instead of taking an all-over shower.

- **Manage your wound dressing.** A number of measures should be taken, including leaving the dressing in place for at least twenty-four hours. After that, the dressing can be replaced with clean, dry gauze if you have significant drainage. If it comes off, leave it off or redress the wound—again, with clean, dry gauze. All dressings should be taken off before taking a shower. Use soap and water in the shower, but don't scrub the wound. Pat the area dry—don't rub it dry—after getting out of the shower. Then replace the dressing.

- **Take care with sutures.** For the most part, sutures to close wounds will absorb into your tissues. However, some may need to be removed at the surgeon's office a week or two following your procedure. Occasionally, small openings may appear along an incision site, and these require additional attention such as washing with soap and water, applying an antibiotic cream, or more frequent redressing. Check with your surgeon for proper care procedures. A suture abscess is an area of drainage related to the suture, which can often look infected. Fortunately, they tend to resolve once they drain.

- **Elevation is key.** Sleeping propped up against a pillow to elevate your face after a facelift is extremely important. Elevation helps dramatically to reduce swelling and discomfort, especially when dealing with extremities.

- **Be active, but not too active too soon.** In short, if any activity causes significant pain, don't do it. Moderate walking is encouraged, but strenuous activity or heavy lifting should be avoided following a procedure. Early ambulation is associated with a quicker recovery and fewer postoperative complications.

- **Compression.** Many types of cosmetic plastic surgery procedures require some type of compression during healing: liposuction, skin excisions, tummy tuck, chin lift, and others. Compression helps control swelling and inflammation and improves comfort. Think about when you bump your head— the first thing you do is reach up and rub the point of impact. When you do that, it feels better—because you're applying pressure. Among the compression options are wraps, such as ACE bandages, which are a good choice because they are so versatile. They adjust to individual body sizes and differences; immediately following surgery, there is not typically a lot of swelling, but within a few days, there tends to be quite a bit more due to the body's inflammatory response. Another option is to order garments off the internet that can be downsized as time passes, the swelling subsides, and your body adjusts to its new size. Basically, they can be reduced by about 20 percent per week. However, the challenge of the prefit garments is that everyone is different, so they tend to fit tight on one part of the body and loose somewhere else. It can be a little tricky to find garments that are comfortable everywhere; instead, often these make the healing process a little more miserable for most people.

Ultimately, it's going to take time to heal. Tissue is dynamic; it changes with time, both through the healing process and the swelling and scarring. It's not an absolute or exact science, but depending on the patient, there is a typical timeline for healing.

The Day of Surgery

After the surgery, you may not experience much pain because it takes time for the anesthesia to wear off, and you may be on other pain medications. In fact, it's not uncommon to feel really great immediately after a cosmetic plastic surgery procedure. This may be due to the body's fight-or-flight stress response—it's a little like being in an accident; immediately after you're typically in a very excited state.

Although there is not always a lot of swelling right away, the swelling can have a rapid onset and increase dramatically in size over the first twenty-four to seventy-two hours after surgery. As I mentioned earlier, there is also a considerable amount of fluid drainage postsurgery, which appears reddish or watery in nature.

Postsurgery, we really want patients to ambulate at least three times a day for twenty minutes or so each time. As mentioned, early ambulation is key to preventing many perioperative anesthetic and procedure complications.

Day One Postprocedure

The first day after surgery or a procedure is when most people begin to see the onset of really significant swelling along with an increase in discomfort and pain.

While you may not have much appetite at this point, it's essential to hydrate—fluids are essential to preventing dehydration.

Again, we also want patients to ambulate multiple times during the day. The last thing we want is for you to lie down on the couch and stay there for a week. Movement can help prevent deep vein thrombosis, or blood clots in the legs that can translate to the lungs. Moving around also helps with pulmonary respiration to prevent pneumonia.

Often, the first day postsurgery the patient actually still feels pretty great—but that's a false indicator of how the healing journey is going to be.

Day Two Postprocedure

The second day after surgery or a procedure there can be a dramatic reversal of that first-day great feeling. Patients often feel like they've been "hit by a truck" on this day—this is very normal at this point following many procedures. That's often because of fatigue but also potentially part of that fight-or-flight response—again, like being in a car wreck, you really start to feel it a day or two later.

Especially with something like liposuction, swelling significantly increases at this point, particularly compared to the baseline rate after the procedure. Drainage, however, usually begins to slow at this time.

One Week Postprocedure

A week after surgery or a procedure, any drains placed can typically be removed. Patients may experience hyper- or hyposensation in the areas of surgery, meaning they may have some extreme sensitivity or extreme numbness. Incisions can become irritated or even open in small areas. In chapter 7, I talk all about the actual healing process, including what is happening when an incision opens or gaps and what should be done about it.

Three Weeks Postprocedure

This is a crucial point in the healing process. Under normal circumstances, at three weeks, it is difficult and unlikely that there will be a problem with a wound that has healed, and it's unlikely that the incision can be injured. Any bandages or wound-closure strips still remaining are typically removed by this point in time.

At three weeks, incisions often look great, and scars are thin because it is early on in the healing process. If the incisions are closed and healed, patients can begin scar management with silicone tape or gel.

HEALING TIMELINE

- Three weeks: Adequate wound strength

- Six weeks: Unrestricted activity

- Three months: Breast surgery has settled

- Six months: Swelling resolves for liposuction

- One year: The earliest point at which scarring has improved

- Two years: Maximal neurogenic function returns

Oftentimes, areas that may not have been painful after surgery now become tender and may experience neurogenic pain, a shooting, burning, tingling type pain that is a result of nerve function. This can increase in severity over a couple of weeks but will plateau and eventually go away.

Six Weeks Postprocedure

Most people can return to unrestricted activity prior to this point in the healing process. Activity levels are adjusted based on individual patients and procedures. Six weeks is also when most folks can stop wearing compression or cut back on wearing it if they choose. This is also the point where most patients ask, "Is this how it's going to look?" Again, we remind patients that the healing is not nearly complete at this point.

Three Months Postprocedure

Three months is how long it takes for breast surgery—an augmentation or lift—to settle in and assume the new position and size.

At three months, scars can become worse or appear to worsen. They may become redder or thicker; they may widen and become raised. They may actually worsen even more over the next few months, especially compared to the initial healing.

Six Months Postprocedure

This is when liposuction and skin-tightening procedures reach their maximum improvement. In general, this is also the earliest that any type of revision or additional procedure to the area can be done.

One Year Postprocedure

This is the average time that it takes for scars to improve to their maximal result. It's also the earliest that revisional surgery can be done to the nose after a rhinoplasty.

At one year, any fluctuation swelling should be subsiding. Fluctuation swelling occurs after procedures such as abdominoplasty (tummy tucks). For the first year, patients may notice that their belly or abdomen is flat in the morning but swollen by the end of the day. That's due to gravity and the inability of fluid to cross over the scar at the bottom of the abdomen. It takes one year at a minimum for the lymphatic channels to be established and function properly.

Two Years Postprocedure

This is how long it takes for nerve function to fully resolve and for maximal return of sensation. Areas that are numb at two years most likely will remain numb.

❖ ❖ ❖

The family role in this process is extremely important and often underestimated. It's natural for human beings in general to try to minimize risks and the difficulties that can be encountered during recovery. That's one reason it's crucial to have the family involved from the beginning.

Again, one of the problems that we often see is that family members do not always agree with the patient's desire to have a procedure done, or they may not always understand why they're doing it. But the patient truly needs to try to get family support, because the more the family understands, ideally, the more supportive they will be.

Too often, the family doesn't understand how impactful their role is during the recovery, and they need to be brought in early on if they're going to play a major role in the recovery. They need to be aware of that role because negative opinions or offhand comments like "You shouldn't have done this" or "You look worse than you did before" do not help the patient's emotional well-being during recovery. Nothing constructive comes out of that kind of attitude or "help." The patient's family needs to be prepared to be supportive during recovery, and if they're not going to be, then the patient will probably need to find somebody else to help them postsurgery, or they may need to decide whether to do the surgery. In chapter 8, I share some tips for talking to family early on about their upcoming role.

Unfortunately, what happens too often with surgery in general is that the infamous out-of-town or uninvolved family member shows up at a post-op visit with a stern look on their face and upset that their family member's recovery isn't going as it should without having any understanding of what's gone on. They haven't been in on the consultation; they don't know what's been discussed. There's almost a savior mentality by that family member who shows up and is going to fix everything now because the patient's either unhappy or the recovery is not going as well or as quickly as they thought it would. But all that does is drive a wedge between the patient and doctor, and in some ways, other family members because then they feel more justified in saying, "You shouldn't have done this" or "Look what you did to yourself." But without being involved, they don't understand that when it's only three or six weeks after surgery, the patient is not supposed to love how they look yet. That's one reason we really want to start the dialogue with everyone early and that we recommend counseling for everyone involved.

When family isn't involved from the beginning, they often cause problems by feeding misinformation to the patient or bringing up someone else's experience that has nothing to do with this particular case. Once that starts, it becomes almost impossible for the doctor-patient relationship to have trust and to continue to nurture the patient's recovery. I call this the Aunt-Betty-Said syndrome, which I talk more about in chapter 9.

Cosmetic plastic surgery is a journey that can involve the entire family, before, during, and especially after the procedure. It's crucial that everyone understands the process and knows that it takes patience to get final results. Outcomes generally improve with time.

"I WAS ALWAYS
LOOKING OUTSIDE
MYSELF FOR STRENGTH
AND CONFIDENCE,
BUT IT COMES FROM
WITHIN. IT IS THERE
ALL THE TIME."

—ANNA FREUD

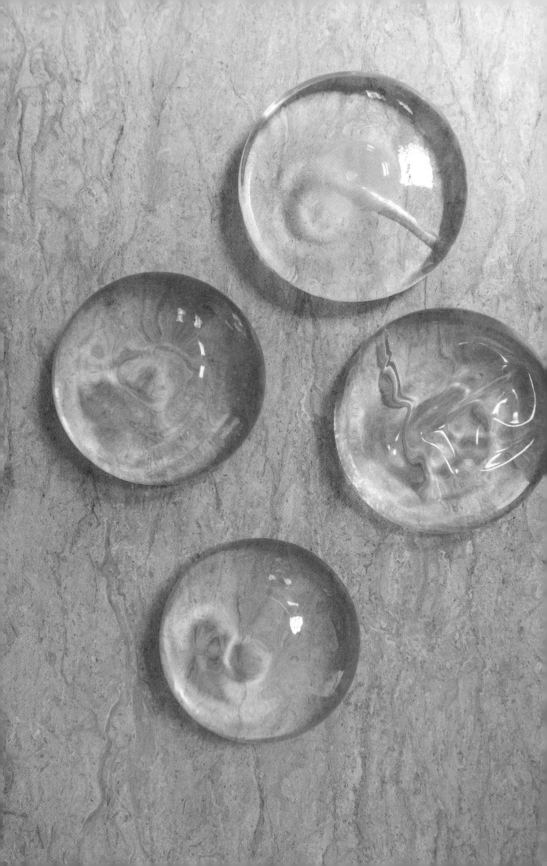

CHAPTER 6

"Tell Me What I Need; You're the Expert"

YOU'RE THE PLASTIC SURGEON; TELL ME WHAT I NEED FIXED.

When Sara came to my practice for a consult, I asked, "What can I help you with?"

She replied, "Well, you're the expert; tell me what I need done." I cannot tell you how many times a patient has sat across from me in a consult and made that statement, followed by, "If I were your wife or family member, what would you tell me to do?"

As many people can, I, too, can certainly see some of the effects that childbearing and gravity have had on a woman's body. I can certainly see how aging is beginning to show in a man's or woman's face. As a plastic surgeon, I can identify areas of the body that I believe are improvable through surgery or other procedures. But what I may observe about a person's body, what that person may observe, and what other people may observe can be completely different.

My role is to take a generalized insecurity and drill down to specifics. So if a patient is unhappy with her skin, for example, I try to determine exactly where the unhappiness lies: Is it the loss of volume? The excess wrinkles? The discoloration of the skin? I won't just look at a patient and tell her what needs to be done. I have to figure out specifically what's bothering her and determine whether the procedures, surgeries, and processes that we have are safe for her and are going to address her concerns so she will be happy. For instance, when Leesa came to see me, I thought when I first entered the consultation room that she had come to see me about the excess skin around her eyes. But when I asked what I could do for her, she said she wanted something done about the sagging skin on her neck. So from an expert point of view, I felt that her eyes were making her look older. But what was making her unhappy was seeing her mother's double chin in the mirror.

As I tell other patients who do not know what they want, I told Sara that we offer many different procedures that can improve a variety of different issues. But if I were to perform ten procedures on a patient and none of them really targeted what the patient wanted, that patient would never be happy with anything I've done. That goes for any plastic surgeon. I can honestly say having an unhappy, discontented patient is an emotional drain on the surgeon and the whole practice. We take patients' opinions and outcomes personally. No one wants a patient to be happy with the outcome more than I do, so it is paramount to align a patient's goals and expectations with the procedure's most likely outcome as well as the possibility of challenges or delays in the healing process.

There are common procedures that can help people, depending on their situations. A "mommy makeover," for instance, can help enhance areas of the body such as the breasts and tummy after pregnancy. But the face, for instance, is one area that is very subjective: people's perceptions of their faces are unique to them. Few other people will see the same things.

If people want a procedure to help them look more rested, there are absolutely some good, straightforward options. Blepharoplasty (eyelid surgery), for instance, is a simple procedure that helps to correct sagging and drooping eyelid skin that comes with aging. It can also correct chronic puffiness below the eyes due to herniating fat pads, which can make a person look very tired. Often, patients tell me their coworkers, friends, or family members have told them they look tired or angry. Eyelid surgery is a great option for men and women who want to regain a more youthful appearance. It is an affordable procedure that comes with little to no risk, and requires very minimal recovery time—typically three to five days—yet it can dramatically improve how awake and healthy a person looks.

As I mentioned in chapter 3, there are some very good, affordable skin-resurfacing options that have little or no downtime. Skin resurfacing decreases the size of pores, improves or treats sun damage, and gives the patient a rested, improved appearance. In short, the skin glows and overall looks healthier. Many skin-resurfacing options work because they stimulate collagen and elastin, tightening skin. Skin-resurfacing options include skin peels and dermabrasions, which help tighten skin to smooth out wrinkles while eliminating sunspots and brown spots. Another option, laser resurfacing, uses pulsating beams of light or energy to correct wrinkles and scars on irregular skin. Microneedling, or micro-ablative treatment, is a system that pierces the skin to naturally stimulate collagen production, which reduces wrinkles and improves skin texture. A CO_2 laser treatment device uses micropulses of energy to rejuvenate skin and give it a smoother look. Skin-resurfacing options are ideal for people who don't want to look as if they have "had something done." The procedure can be done on a Thursday or Friday, and you can be back at work on Monday looking refreshed and rejuvenated but not overdone. Most recently, radiofrequency (RF) microneedling is gaining great traction in the cosmetic world. This procedure uses microneedles to transmit heat, causing fat to melt and skin to contract and tighten. The results thus far with the advancements in this technology show great promise and entail minimal downtime.

These are the kinds of procedures I suggest as options for people who are unsure of what they want. As I mentioned earlier, I really have to drill down on the specifics of what makes people unhappy and match the source of their unhappiness or discontent with procedures that can deliver reasonable results. Some patients come to a consult with little more than the feeling that they "look old," which takes some considerable discussion. I have to ask what the patient means by "look old": whether the patient thinks their skin looks unhealthy because of exposure to the sun, or they have unwanted wrinkles or areas of unwanted, saggy skin.

Such questions represent the kind of exploratory questions a plastic surgeon should ask. It is not the place of plastic surgeons to point out anyone's imperfections. Instead, they should ask questions and listen carefully to the answers to get a better understanding of the issues that are important to the patient and thus determine which areas to improve.

Once a conversation begins, many patients open up because they know what results they are after. But some are hesitant to share their thoughts, even with a plastic surgeon who is there to help them. They may actually be embarrassed to ask for help. Some even apologize. "I'm so sorry you have to see this," they may say. While some people do have serious issues, most just have an overly negative view of themselves. I and my staff are not there to judge. Our role is to help determine whether patients can have a good outcome and whether they will be pleased with their results. I don't compare patients to some predefined standard of body perfection. The goal is to discover what the best procedure will be for each individual. The patient deserves an individualized treatment plan tailored to their specific desires, physical baseline, and goals. I've even seen wives turn away from their husbands to show me something they "never let him see." Believe me, if you are that embarrassed about something on your body, you deserve credit for taking the initiative to make a change.

> It is not the place of plastic surgeons to point out anyone's imperfections. Instead, they should ask questions and listen carefully to the answers to get a better understanding of the issues that are important to the patient and thus determine which areas to improve.

I think a patient's hesitation may be driven by intimidation or even media hype because I'm often asked if I look at people and immediately decide what they "need" done. It's true that most employees in a plastic surgery office are good representations of what plastic surgery can offer. Most have had one or more procedures done, so they tend to be ambassadors. And of course, plastic surgeons have a reputation in the media for trying to "create perfection." So, whether in the office or on the street, it seems that people I meet often wonder whether they are being judged. I can assure you that we do not do that—the only thing that matters to me is a patient's happiness, and that can only be achieved by improving what they see in themselves and what they want to improve.

I try to assess people's issues, ensure they understand what can and can't be done, and have realistic expectations of the outcome. I then find potential treatments and procedures that will ideally meet their desired goals. Connecting with the patient and building a level of trust is part of what can determine whether a patient has a good overall experience. When a patient has an unhappy plastic surgery experience, it is often not from the lack of having the procedure explained, or from a lack of preparation by the plastic surgeon and team. It is often an issue of comprehension: the instructions about a procedure or recovery may not have been completely understood, or the patient's expectations may not have been realistic. Patients who comprehend what a procedure can deliver, have realistic expectations about outcomes, and follow the surgeon's orders for recovery tend to have far better experiences overall.

I can't overemphasize how much we want to avoid unhappy, discontented patients at my practice. Unhappy patients are an emotional and professional drain on my staff and me. And it's unfortunate that their unhappiness usually comes from an outside force—other family members, friends, associates, people who are "experts." At times, outside influences—nonmedical influences—can even build animosity between the patient and the surgeon. They may even say something along the lines of, "My friend said this doesn't look right, so you need to do something about it." It can be frustrating for the doctor to have to defend their medical treatment against someone with no medical experience. The idea that the surgeon is avoiding doing a procedure that would make the healing go faster—should there be such a thing—is categorically wrong. By listening to others, often out of the belief that their nonmedical advisers have their best interests at heart, patients put their health and their outcomes at risk. But if patients insist they want to see another doctor, I will happily help them find a qualified, experienced surgeon as a second opinion.

Again, it's important to also remember the role family members play postoperatively, that patients are vulnerable and emotionally drained after surgery and that relationships established in advance with counselors can be invaluable to patients and family both before and after surgery. In spite of a stigma about counseling, in my practice, we encourage you to consider it before surgery so that you have that connection before any stressors occur after the procedure.

When it comes to cosmetic plastic surgery, the best course of action is to follow a checklist:

- decide you want something done for you

- be very thorough in assessing and researching potential offices and doctors

- get buy-in from your spouse, family, friends, and anyone else who can give you support

- commit to the process

- be fair to the process, allowing adequate time for results to be achieved

I have come to realize, and often jokingly tell patients, that "patience is not the American way." People want immediate results, and postoperative recovery is not an immediate process. In addition, everyone views themselves as different—the exception. Often, I tell a patient a routine healing course is four to six weeks, and they respond by saying, "I am a quick healer." Two weeks later, they are in the office complaining about not being healed and back to normal. Their perception is not in line with reality.

With all the variables involved in cosmetic plastic surgery, it can sometimes be helpful to compare plastic surgery procedures to other professional services. For instance, a financial planner who invests a client's money cannot be 100 percent certain of the investment outcome. Instructors cannot predict with complete accuracy what their students will take away from their learning experience and how they will apply it. There are, unfortunately, no true "crystal balls" in life, and there are certainly none in the plastic surgery world.

So as technology continues to advance in improving outcomes and results while decreasing recovery time and challenges, cosmetic plastic surgery remains an art, not an exact science, and there are no absolute guarantees. Still, there are some things to look for that can help improve the overall experience.

A good surgeon–patient relationship. Patients today try to take an active role in their care and treatment. While most patients are very pleasant, understanding, and proactive about the process, other patients can be more challenging. Those patients tend to be the ones whose decision to pursue plastic surgery was driven by emotion. Highly charged emotions can add to the energy of the process, sometimes in negative ways. That is why it is important for you, the patient, to feel comfortable with your plastic surgeon. Open communication can help ensure that you both share the same vision and goals, and your expectations are in line with anticipated outcomes. If you feel your concerns are not being acknowledged and addressed, your surgeon–patient relationship may be too problematic—and that can make the experience extremely difficult after the surgery.

Caring office staff. The office staff should be easy to interact with and responsive, and they should appear to be genuinely compassionate and concerned about you and your family. Office staff who are attuned to the various energies of patients and understand the critical nature of genuine interaction can help reduce the negative energy of patients who are frustrated with their experience. Unfortunately, things are missed in every office at some point. This is unavoidable, but ultimately, the office needs to have the patients' care and satisfaction as its number-one priority.

Experience and confidence. Obviously, you want a plastic surgeon who is well experienced and well trained. You should also work with someone who has the experience and training in the type of procedure you are interested in, someone who performs that procedure on a regular basis. Also ask about the surgeon's volume of procedures, board certification, and how they will handle complications or dissatisfied patients. I try to reassure patients that we will do whatever it takes to make them happy. I view our service as a product and our patients as consumers. Like any business, I believe we need to stand behind our product and ensure patient satisfaction.

"I'm the best" claims. Confidence in a surgeon's ability is a must. However, beware of surgeons who tout that they are the best, the only ones who know what they're doing. Research surgeons who make you feel like they know what they're doing, but not to the point of being obnoxious. An arrogant doctor who is "never wrong" can make for difficult interactions with patients and with other colleagues the patient may need at some point in the care process. "Misplaced pride" actually resulted in a life sentence for a neurosurgeon in Texas, who was convicted of "intentionally causing serious bodily injury" after he continued to operate, even when his procedures led to death or paralysis.[13]

Useful second opinions. Surgeons who unjustly belittle the competition can signal insecurity and an ego that is a challenge to work with—or worse, overcompensation for their skill set. A surgeon who gives alarmist second opinions—"That procedure was incor-

---

13   Deb Jones, "Texas Jury Imposes Life Sentence on Neurosurgeon," *The Daily Voice News*, February 21, 2017, accessed May 6, 2017, http://thedailyvoicenews. com/2017/02/21/texas-jury-imposes-life-sentence-on-neurosurgeon/.

rectly done in the first place!"—can cause a great deal of anxiety for the patient and unwarranted issues for the original surgeon. Second opinions are very useful, but patients need to be educated in the process and understand the dynamics at play. A second opinion from a noncosmetic plastic surgeon—or, perhaps even worse, an urgent care facility—may not necessarily be the best, as this is not their area of expertise, because that surgeon likely specializes primarily in reconstructive surgery. In most institutional settings, little or no cosmetic plastic surgery is performed. So while the opinions may be valid for reconstructive issues, when it comes to cosmetic plastic procedures, you are relying on the input of someone who does not perform that kind of work on a regular basis. Certainly, unforeseen things can happen. Second opinions are great as long as they're from a qualified, reputable, and experienced provider with broad experience in the area in question. Otherwise, you're just throwing more gas on the fire.

We see a lot of patients who have consulted with other plastic surgeons first before choosing us for their procedures. When a patient comes to me after having an unhappy experience with another plastic surgeon, I prefer to look ahead to what can be achieved instead of reliving the drama the patient may have already been through. Being critical of another surgeon to somehow increase my own value to a patient is not productive. "Your experience is unfortunate," I tell such patients. "Now let's look at what we can do to get you where you want to be." That little bit of compassion can lead to a relationship resulting in a beautiful cosmetic plastic surgery experience.

I am amazed at how patients and their families will latch on to opinions they want to hear: "My primary care doctor says my wound is infected." While I respect all opinions from other physicians and surgeons, contradictory opinions from physicians or surgeons who have never performed the same surgery are not helpful and can cause animosity between the patient and the surgeon who performed the procedure. There is a reason why there are subspecialties within medicine. The complexities associated with surgery are many, and postoperative management is best done by the surgeon experienced in the preoperative assessment of a patient, the performance of the surgical procedure, and the postoperative management of such procedures. As a surgeon, I only want the best outcome possible for my patient and will do anything possible to ensure that.

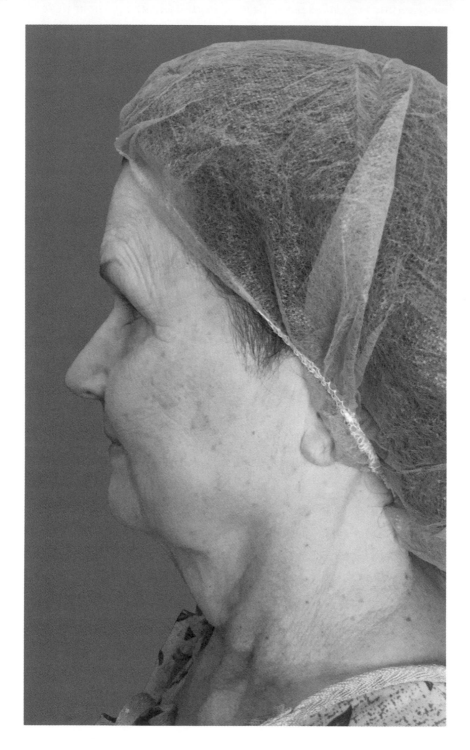

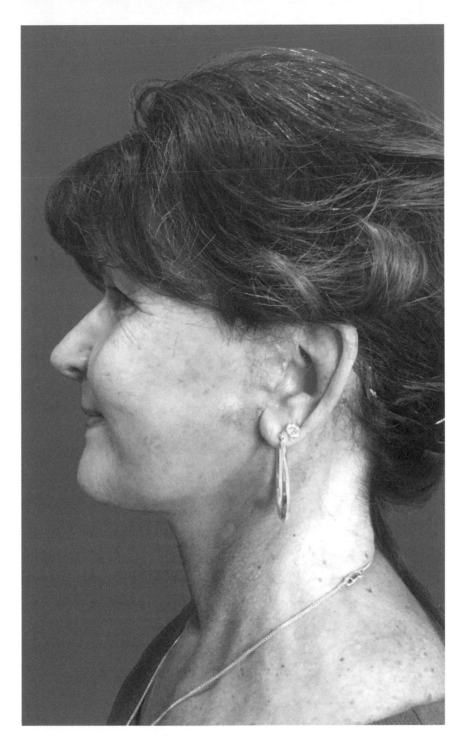

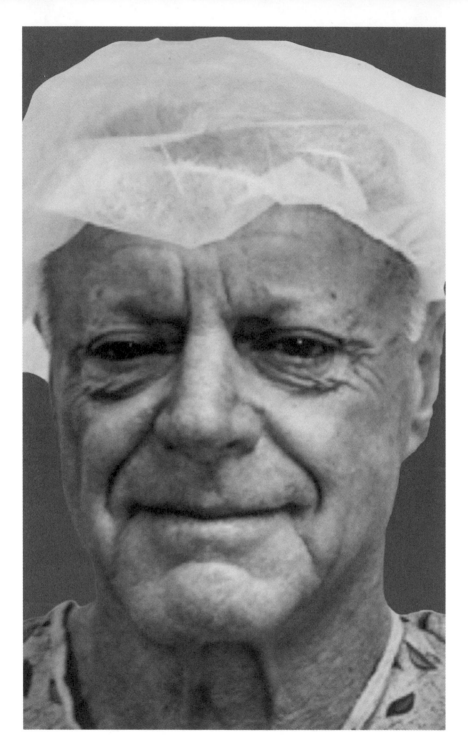

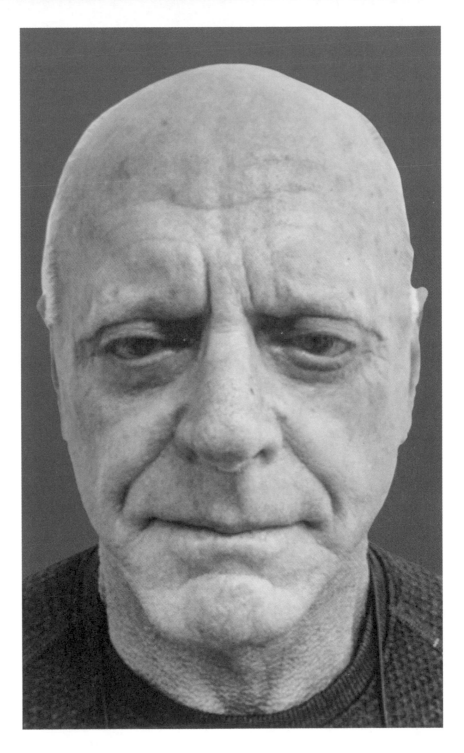

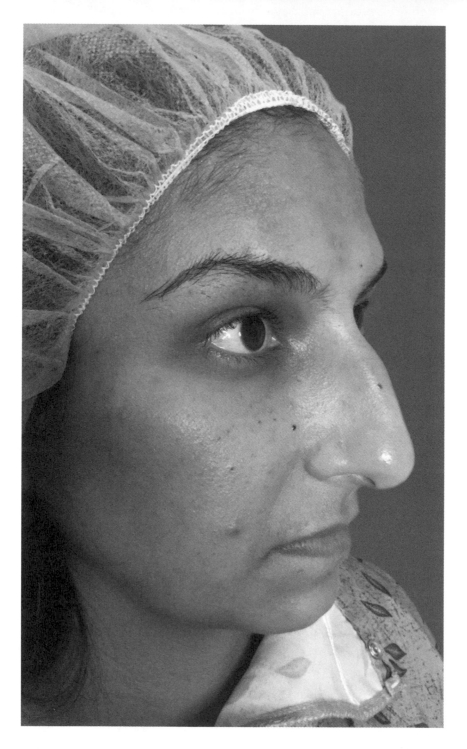

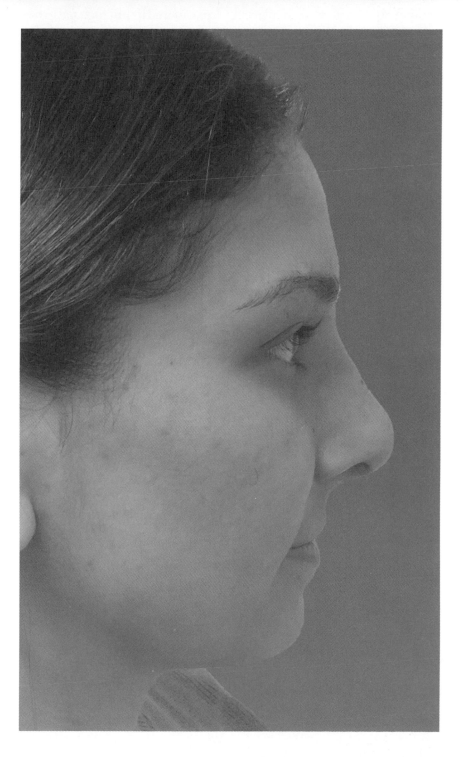

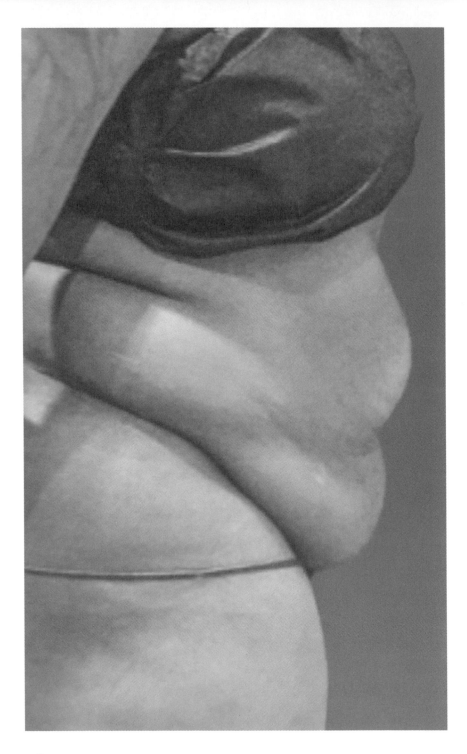

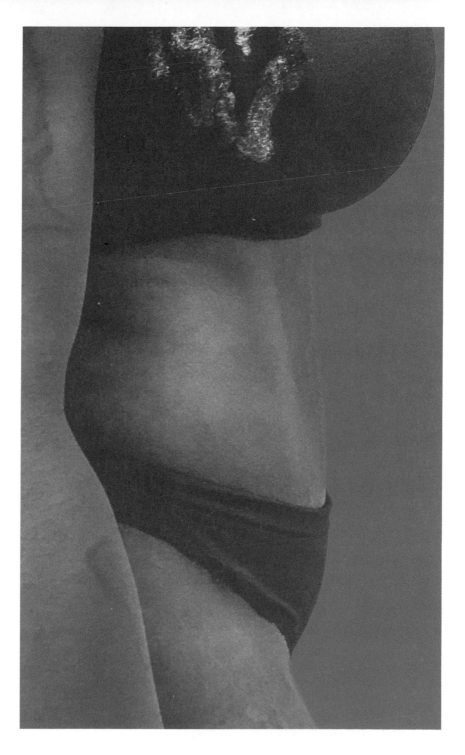

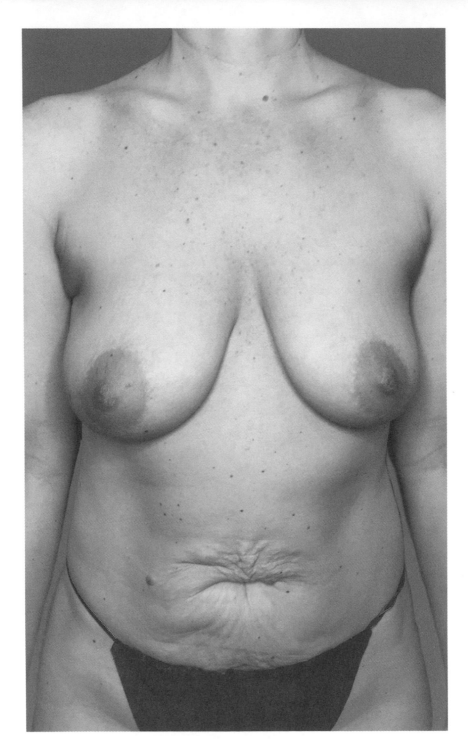

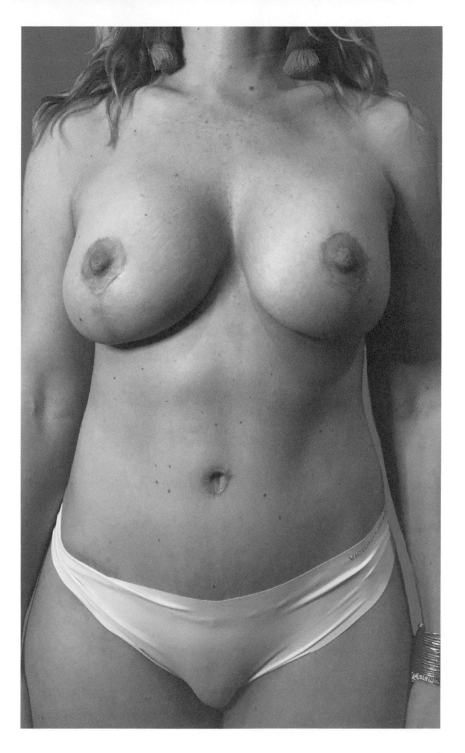

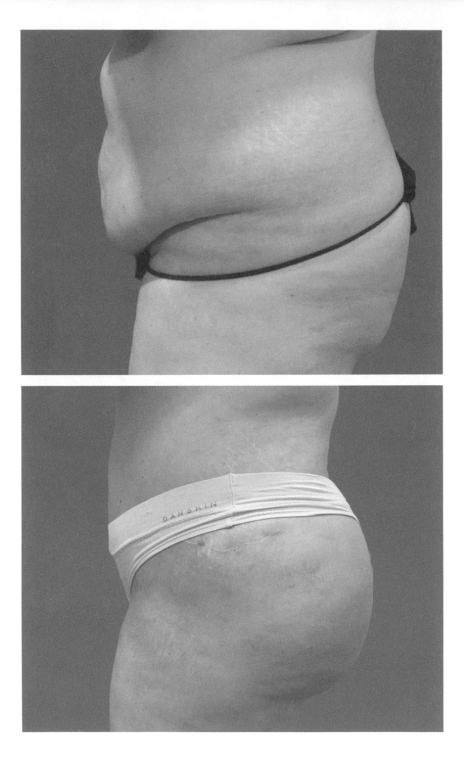

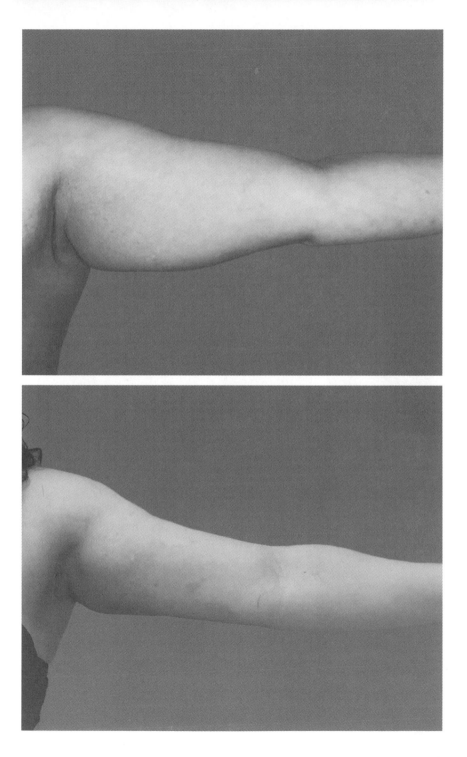

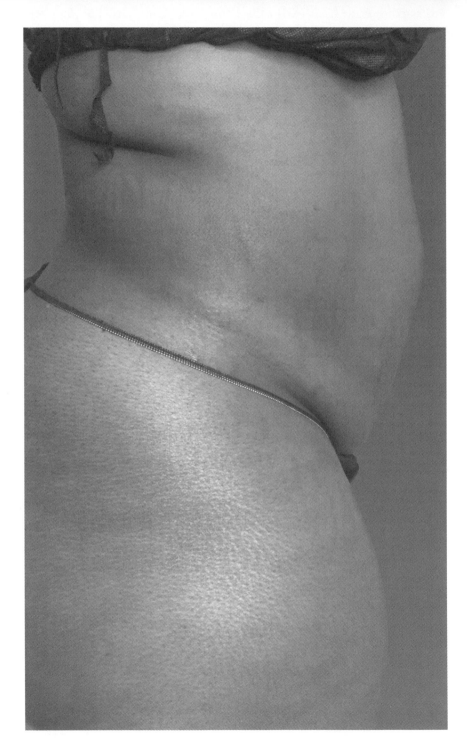

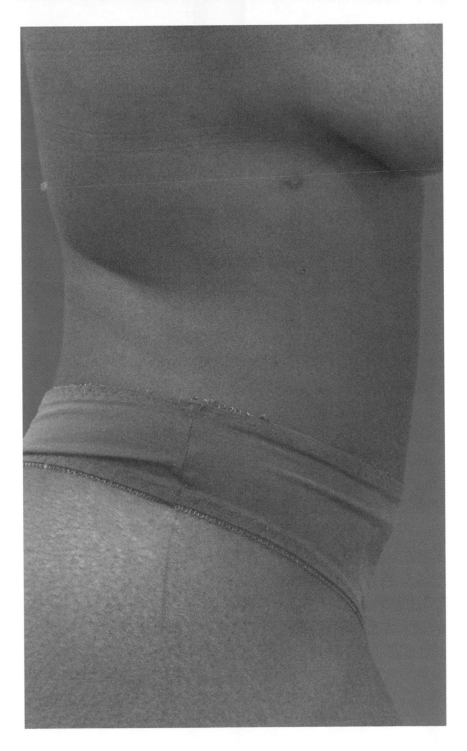

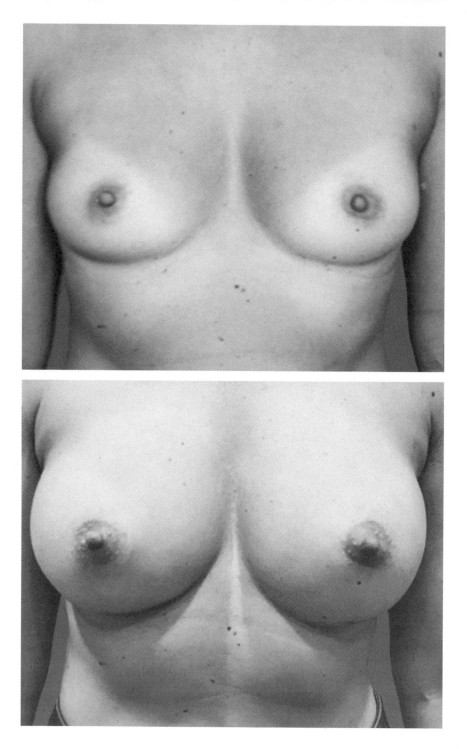

"WE ARE
WHAT WE BELIEVE
WE ARE."

—C.S. LEWIS

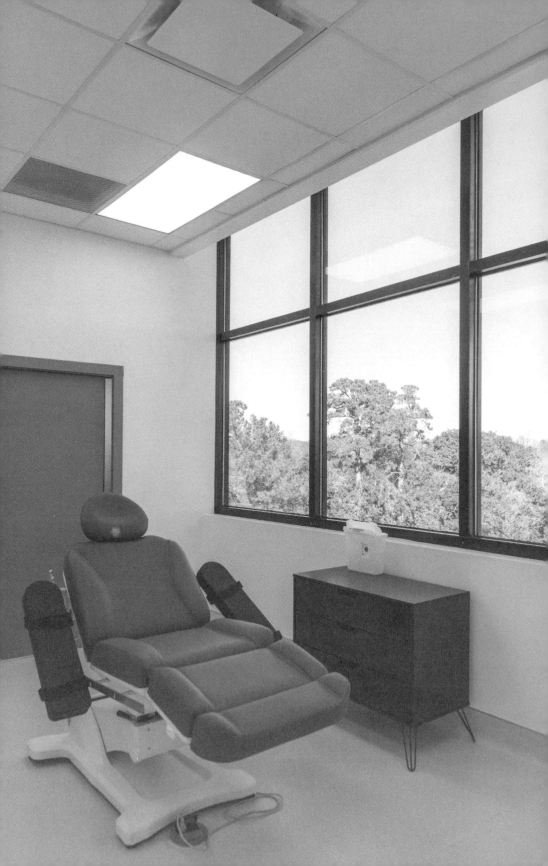

CHAPTER 7

"I Want to Look More Like ... "

HOW LONG WILL IT TAKE TO HAVE A "NEW ME"?

Since patients come from all walks of life, the plastic surgeon must learn how to relate to a wide range of cultural, financial, and educational backgrounds. An approach that works to build trust with one patient may be completely different from what works with another. I do believe relatability is a crucial factor that leads to an open, honest, and trustworthy relationship between the patient and surgeon.

For instance, most patients are not ultrarich, and they run the gamut of professions. At my practice, we see young professionals who are in the early stages of their careers and want breast augmentation, Botox, or a nose job—something they've wanted for years. We have single women and men who are midway through their careers and have a steady job and are out on the social scene. Especially here in the South, people spend a lot of time outdoors, so they want to look good in shorts and swimsuits. We see moms looking for that "mommy makeover" I mentioned earlier. And we see double-income professionals such as teachers, police officers, firefighters, and members of the military for whom plastic surgery is attainable and achievable, depending on their circumstances. So building a connection with so many different personalities is a welcome challenge.

For the many different types of potential patients with wide-ranging backgrounds, a variety of procedures are available. Especially for someone who is new to plastic surgery, it may be advisable to ease into surgery with a minor procedure: a little Botox, filler, laser skin care, or eyelid surgery. In fact, as I've mentioned, some noninvasive or minimally invasive procedures allow you to return to work in a few days. An eyelid procedure performed on a Friday, for instance, may allow you to return to work the following week with little to no evidence of the procedure, hopefully looking refreshed. The pandemic situation and the number of people working from home and wearing masks became an ideal opportunity for finally getting a procedure done. In fact, the AAFPRS annual survey found that 96 percent of patients were having something done because, due to social distancing and working from home, they had more time and flexibility in their schedules to recover from treatment.[14]

In some ways, it seems to me that plastic surgery unites people, regardless of culture. Wanting to feel good about yourself and having confidence in the way that you look and how you feel, in the way you look in clothing, can lead to a higher level of confidence, no matter your walk of life. Appearance gives you confidence in your job performance;

---

14   "AAFPRS Announces Annual Survey Results: A Look at How Covid-19 Disrupted Facial Plastic Surgery & Aesthetics," news release, February 1, 2021, American Academy of Facial Plastic and Reconstructive Surgery, accessed February 24, 2021, https://www.aafprs.org/Media/Press_Releases/New%20Stats%20AAFPRS%20 Annual%20Survey.aspx.

again, that's especially important in jobs like sales or where you're in the public eye. People in these jobs want to look refreshed and pleasant and be approachable, and that all transcends cultural differences. So, irrespective of cultural background, there is a desire by people to feel good about themselves and how they look and to be accepted by the people around them. With all the things going on in our world that are separating or dividing people, in some ways, cosmetic plastic surgery unites people because we want similar things, irrespective of our backgrounds.

> Wanting to feel good about yourself and having confidence in the way that you look and how you feel, in the way you look in clothing, can lead to a higher level of confidence, no matter your walk of life.

While we have similar objectives—to be accepted and to feel good about ourselves—our perceptions differ along cultural lines about the definition of beauty and how to achieve it. I see that in my practice: people from different cultures want surgery that accomplishes different goals. Certain surgeries are desired more by certain cultures than others.

For example, the procedure known as the Brazilian butt lift or fat grafting to augment the bottom is definitely something that we see requested more by Latin American or African American women, whereas Caucasian women tend to want more fullness in their lips (not their hips).

Although women of all cultures pursue breast augmentation, women from some cultures tend to already naturally have more fullness, so they don't need or want as much out of the procedure.

Age and childbirth are also unifying experiences, irrespective of culture. Childbirth physically changes a woman's body pretty significantly, so we see women from all races and cultures who want something done to help them get back their prebaby bodies, to start feeling like their younger selves before they had children.

Culture can play a role not only in the types of surgeries people want but also in their expectations regarding outcomes. For instance, when we perform liposuction on Latin American or African American women, we're typically asked to leave some curves and fullness, whereas Caucasian women often want more fullness removed during such a procedure.

Latinx and African Americans also tend to have fuller cheek structures, cheekbones, lips, and other features, so they tend to request fewer procedures in these areas, or less aggressive changes from procedures, whereas some Caucasians tend to have weaker facial structures and request more fillers and other procedures to restore volume.

When it comes to scarring and discoloration of the skin, cultural backgrounds make for significant differences. For instance, Latinx and African American people don't have issues with sun exposure and sun damage because the amount of melanin and pigment in their skin tends to help it age better and slower. They don't request skin restoration procedures nearly as often as Caucasians do.

However, some of the challenges with healing skin that is hyperpigmented include keloids, which are aggressive scars that can form a smooth, hard surface that is not harmful but is unattractive. People with darker pigmented skin tend to be more at risk for developing keloid scars.[15]

African American communities also tend to have higher incidences of unaddressed hypertension and diabetes, which can complicate healing from any kind of surgery, including cosmetic plastic

---

15   "Keloid Scar of Skin," Healthline, accessed July 5, 2017, http://www.healthline.com/health/keloids#overview1.

surgery. We want to acknowledge these types of medical risks so we can address them appropriately during treatment.

Scars can vary from patient to patient, and circumstances such as genetics and postsurgical wound management can play a role in how much a person scars.

The location of the incision can also be a factor in how a scar appears. The classic example of how location factors into scarring is when a woman undergoes a Cesarean section (C-section) procedure during childbirth. Often, a C-section scar heals quite well. Why is that? Because when a woman is pregnant, her abdomen skin is extremely stretched. When it is sutured back together during the C-section, the tissue is void of tension, so it just falls back together. Many C-section scars end up as little more than thin lines.

Scarring from cosmetic plastic surgery can be more complicated, since it often involves removing excess tissue or stretching tissue to make it tight and flat. Making the site tight and flat involves placing the tissue under tension—sometimes great tension—to pull it tight and shape it. Those forces can cause scars to be wider and thicker. So while an abdominoplasty (tummy tuck) incision is in the same place as a C-section, since they are created for completely different circumstances, they will heal differently. The reason is that if the tissue is not pulled tightly or stretched at the time of surgery, it will be loose afterward, and the patient will not be happy.

Scars in all patients usually begin as extremely red and raised, with very firm tissue. With any cosmetic plastic surgery, the final results are not immediate. The surgery itself is an intervention that immediately alters the body's structures. But that alteration is not the final result, and the process, obviously, takes time. Over time, scar tissue will soften and reshape, and its color, texture, and prominence will begin to improve.

While healing begins immediately for most procedures, it can take four to six weeks at a minimum to really begin to see the first results. Healing time varies, depending on the patient. Even though many patients claim they usually heal quickly—and some do have the good fortune of recovering faster than others—the majority of patients take weeks or months to fully heal.

> With any cosmetic plastic surgery, the final results are not immediate.

The amount of time it takes for a person to heal depends on a number of factors, including the specific procedure that was performed, postoperative care, and the person's age and health.

Some procedures can take up to three to six months for results to really be evident. And scars can take up to a year to fully improve. Postabdominoplasty swelling can take one to two years for the reestablishment of the lymphatic system and full resolution of gravity-dependent swelling and bloating.

Throughout recovery, when the incision or wound is healing, it goes through three stages, known as inflammation, proliferation, and maturation. During the inflammation stage, the site swells, making the tissue appear firm, and the patient may experience pain and redness. This first stage can appear as if the healing process is not progressing as it should. In fact, the swelling and redness are usually good signs indicating that the blood vessels in the area are allowing in nutrients, antibodies, enzymes, and white blood cells to stave off infection and promote good healing. The second stage, the proliferation or rebuilding stage, is when new tissue begins to form. In the early days of proliferation, the wound may secrete liquids that can be easy to mistake as infection. In a healthy wound, these liquids are actually part of the healing process to help strengthen and rebuild the area. Finally, the third stage, known as maturation or remodeling, is when the dermal tissues (the skin) gain additional strength. Although the wound may appear to be fully healed when maturation begins, it can take up to two years for maturation of a wound to be complete. In other words, a scar will continue to improve in appearance, texture, and color for twelve to twenty-four months after the procedure, depending on the skin type and genetics of the patient.

Factors that can lengthen healing time include whether a person experiences postsurgery challenges. For instance, sometimes sutured incisions gap, especially where very tight tissue was pulled together to create the suture. Typically, these wounds require little more than extra home care. They do not require resuturing the site.

Gravity can also have an effect on healing tissue. For instance, gravity is an integral part of the healing process after breast augmentation. Initially, breast implants are placed high in the chest, where they are partially covered by muscle and fully covered by skin. That is a necessary part of the procedure because postsurgery, when the patient becomes active, the forces of gravity pull the tissue down, and the implants settle into a more natural position. Some settling occurs in the first six to eight weeks, but it can take up to three months for outcomes after breast augmentation to be fully realized. Breast implants that appear to be in the right place on day five after the surgery will be positioned far too low at the three-month point.

Time is the best cure. Plastic surgery scars usually improve over nine months to a year. Once the skin has become as soft as possible, there are procedures that can improve the scar's appearance including laser treatments, steroid injections, topical tape, creams and lotions, and other management techniques. After the site has fully healed, the scar can sometimes be removed and sutured again. Since that procedure involves only the upper layer of the skin and the scar, and there is no longer tension on the deeper soft-tissue structure, swelling usually does not recur, and healing tends to be much better.

Some of the measures to improve scarring include the following:

- silicone strips
- steroid injections
- the use of a skin pen
- laser treatment; both ablative (i.e., CO2) and non-ablative lasers can be used independently or in conjunction with each other
- scar revision or excision of the scar with closure

For some patients, of course, adjustments may need to be made after healing is complete. In fact, up to 25 percent of the most common procedures, including breast augmentation, need some sort of adjustment in the first two years.[16] The most common reason is that scar tissue has hardened and tightened, forming what's known as a capsular contracture. But making an adjustment while a person is still healing is a little like trying to hit a moving target: it is far more difficult to achieve the expected outcome. With breast procedures, for instance, where symmetry is important, it is best to wait until the tissues have settled completely. Immediately following the surgery, the breasts will appear oversized and even somewhat misshapen. Why is that? Because immediately following surgery, the tissue is traumatized. The breasts will remain swollen for at least several weeks, but over time, they will settle and take on the normal shape. In fact, it takes three months on average for breasts to take on the shape they will settle into.

In spite of the preoperative consult, many patients return for their postoperative visit expressing concerns. For most, all it takes

---

16   N. A. Forster et al., "The Reoperation Cascade after Breast Augmentation with Implants: What the Patient Needs to Know," *Journal of Plastic, Reconstructive & Aesthetic Surgery*, vol. 66, No. 3 (March 2013):313–322; US National Library of Medicine National Institutes of Health, accessed on August 13, 2017, https://www. ncbi.nlm.nih.gov/m/pubmed/23102610/.

is a reminder about all that was discussed prior to the surgery along with the reassurance that the end result cannot be based on what the patient sees the first few days following surgery. The best is yet to come, and if similar cases are any indicator—and they are—the patient will see improvement and have happy outcomes in the weeks and months to come. Again, please be patient.

While there are some issues that should be addressed with your surgeon—significant swelling, drainage, pain, or redness at the surgical site—the bottom line is that healing after most procedures is just going to take time, and that is universal, regardless of culture or genetics.

The better you understand the process prior to the procedure, the less anxiety you will experience postprocedure. During the period of change and healing after surgery, it's easy for patients to obsess about their wounds and about the process. When you're looking at anything on a daily basis, it's very difficult to assess change and see improvements. It's a little like watching paint dry. When you don't see any significant change, it can be frustrating. But when we see patients in our office for appointments that are a few weeks apart, we can clearly see the improvements. In the end, obsessing over healing that is going to take months and that the patient can't do anything about just ends up being a lot of unnecessary anxiety—and that isn't going to help healing.

Trust the process. I've performed thousands of procedures on people from all walks

> **Trust the process.**

of life, so I know that the human body is highly predictable in many ways. In broad terms, bodies heal very similarly, regardless of culture, which is why outcomes are predictable and can be assessed based on averages, although there will always be outliers.

After surgery, it's important to be patient and allow the healing process to occur and the final result to be achieved once the healing is completed.

Becoming a "new you" is a journey. One way to help the journey along is to have "before" pictures on hand. Patients are always amazed when they look back and see "before" pictures of themselves; after they've gone through a procedure, they often forget what they looked like beforehand. During the recovery process, it's good to have those pictures on hand to help both the patient—and family members—have that recall. It's good to keep reminding yourself of where your journey started and how far you have come. That's a great way to help yourself when you feel like things aren't going as you thought they would because, again, healing takes time.

But ideally, once you're finished with your recovery, then you will have more self-confidence, you'll be more outgoing, and you'll be more motivated to get out and do things and enjoy them. After cosmetic plastic surgery, patients who were once reserved and insecure often dress differently, they may be more active and outgoing, and they may have an entirely different attitude because of their new outlook. That may be surprising, unusual, or even difficult for others to understand, especially spouses or significant others, who may even feel threatened by the "new you."

That's why communication with others is important—it's crucial for others to understand what you're going through. It's not entirely uncommon for people who are happy with their outcomes to consider additional procedures—that starts the process all over again with getting family on board and all the prep before and for after the procedure. But when you're happy with your outcome and more com-fortable with your new self, when your family and others see that you did it for the right reasons—to help bring to the surface that inner beauty—then everyone will see that the procedure was a success, and they'll be more confident and understanding of your new you.

"BUT ONE OF THE
BIG LESSONS I HAVE
LEARNED FROM MY
JOURNEY IS YOU CAN'T
PLEASE EVERYONE,
SO DON'T TRY."

—CHRIS COLFER

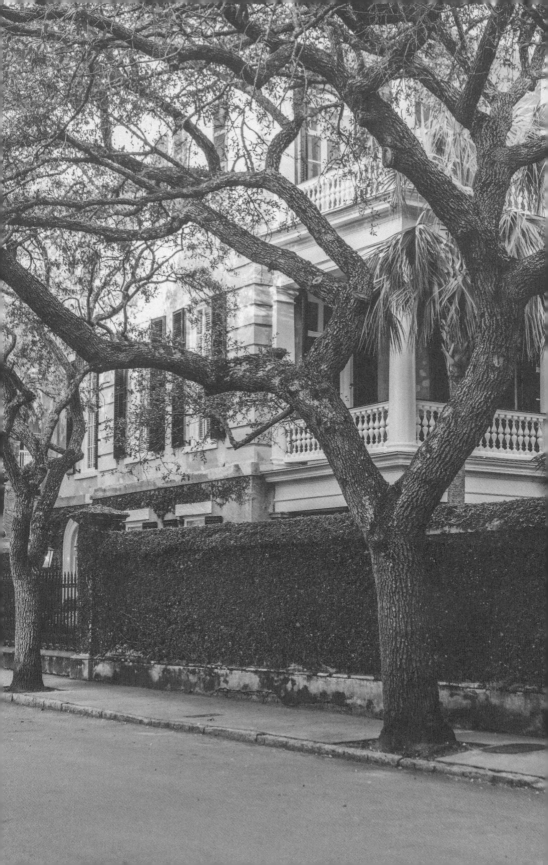

CHAPTER 8

"She Is Already Perfect the Way She Is"

I DON'T UNDERSTAND WHY SHE WANTS TO DO THIS. SHE DOESN'T NEED ANYTHING DONE.

W hen Jill came to me for a consultation, she brought along her husband, Joe. The couple had only been married about a year, but they both had achieved career success and now had some disposable income.

Jill had specific ideas about what she wanted: breast augmentation, or a "boob job." I began by explaining the minimal risks along with the benefits of such a procedure. These days, new shapes and methods for breast implants allow for truly natural-looking results. Most women who undergo the procedure find that their "boob job" helps them feel more confident, feminine, and happy—in and out of their clothing. In the southeastern United States, where we have plenty of beaches and boating, that can be a real plus.

After hearing about the options available and discussing the procedure in depth, Jill turned to Joe and asked, "What do you think, honey?" Joe just looked a little sheepish and shrugged. So in an attempt to ensure he understood everything I had explained, I asked him, "Joe, do you have any questions?" That's when Joe looked up at me and said, "If this is what she wants, OK, but I don't know why she wants it. I love her the way she is. She doesn't need this."

I commonly hear statements like Joe's when discussing a possible cosmetic plastic procedure with a patient whose significant other is present at the discussion. Approximately 80 percent of new patients come to their first consult alone. However, a large majority will bring their spouse or partner to a second visit to finalize the surgical plan and complete preoperative paperwork.

Women especially are likely to be told by their spouse/significant other that they don't "need" cosmetic plastic surgery. "I think she's perfect the way she is," I often hear from the man when a couple comes in prior to her surgery. Some husbands and boyfriends don't realize that a woman's desire for cosmetic plastic surgery goes beyond wanting to impress him. It can be hard for a man to grasp that a woman's desire to improve her looks may have nothing to do with him. Having witnessed so many men say something along the lines of "She doesn't need this procedure to look better," I finally reached out to a psychologist friend of mine, Brian Sullivan, PhD, to better understand what I was hearing. He has worked with many people through various relationship issues and taught in academic centers. His response was simple yet informative: people, especially men, tend to think everything is about them. As a man, I had to chuckle a little to myself when hearing that. Whether the partner's actions are conscious or not, I believe there is truth to the statement.

When a partner or spouse wants to improve her appearance, the man's first thought is that she is doing it *for him*. So he tells her she doesn't need the procedure because that will somehow make her feel better.

A deeper reason for women to seek cosmetic plastic surgery is that they truly want to do something *for themselves*. Women who want cosmetic plastic surgery often do so out of a desire to improve their self-confidence and happiness. They may be attempting to address an issue due to aging or, as I mentioned earlier, something that has bothered them for years that they have never been able to do anything about because of time, finances, or other commitments—or, in some cases, because their partner told them they did not need the procedure. I can't condone the idea of another person telling an adult, accomplished woman what she does or doesn't need.

> A deeper reason for women to seek cosmetic plastic surgery is that they truly want to do something *for themselves*.

Still, often when digging deeper, I find that although the woman wants to feel and be as beautiful as possible, primarily for her own sake, she also wants her spouse or significant other to be proud of her and happy to be seen with her.

In Jill's case, she had felt physically underdeveloped since she had been a teen, which made her self-conscious about her breasts. Having lived her whole life in warm climates, where bathing suits and sundresses are the norm, she always felt that clothes never quite fit her properly. She had never been entirely comfortable in a bathing suit.

For many women, a lack of confidence or a sense of insecurity goes well beyond a spouse's opinion and often precedes the relationship itself—by decades, in some cases.

Jill and Joe are the perfect example of what often happens when one partner is considering cosmetic surgery. Her desire for change had nothing to do with her new husband. All the pieces of her life were coming together—she was sufficiently established and financially secure—so she could address something that had bothered her for years.

I especially see a similar scenario with older couples these days. At the age of sixty, the wife is finally ready to address something about herself that has bothered her for some time, or she wants to shave off a few years to regain a bit of her youthful appearance. Meanwhile, the husband can't quite understand her concerns. He may wonder why, at the age of sixty, his wife cares what her skin or eyes look like. There are any number of reasons he may be concerned about her undergoing a surgical procedure, including the simple fact that she now wants to change something about herself. The subject can become a point of contention in some relationships, causing the woman to decide that it's just not worth pursuing plastic surgery to satisfy her own desires.

But the following tips for talking with your significant other about plastic surgery may help to get him or her on board with the idea:

- **Involve significant others and family members early, and get their buy-in early, if possible.** Unfortunately, sometimes a patient has little support up front, and when things don't quite go as planned, a spouse or significant other is the first to point fingers: "Well, you chose to have this done. You chose to go to see that doctor. I had nothing to do with this process." Sometimes patients don't want anyone to know they've chosen to undergo the procedure. But it's important for the postoperative support team to be on board early. They should even be brought to the office appointment before the procedure so they also have exposure to the process. Getting a spouse, significant other, family member, or other supporters involved earlier in the process gives them accountability and can alleviate some of their anxiety. But be firm in your decision and the desire to proceed if you feel passionately about it. Have conviction about what you want for yourself, and don't allow others to negatively influence that decision.

- **Stay calm.** Regardless of others' reactions, staying calm while you explain your reasoning for wanting a procedure can help you more effectively get your point across.

- **Explain in simple terms your desire for the procedure or improvement.** Use examples that others can relate to—for example, "When the kids left home, we renovated the house and gave it an updated look. Now I want to do the same for myself."

- **Remind family members how important they are to you:** "Doing this for me will make me be a better person for you and for our family."

- **Ask if family members have questions.** Make a list, if needed, of questions you think they might have, and practice your answers in advance. Be prepared to answer others' concerns without getting defensive.

- **Give credence to their opinions.** Allow others to have input into the procedure—the size of implants, for instance, or choice of doctor. When they feel their opinion is valued, they will feel more like part of the process. Ultimately, it is your decision as the patient, but giving value to others' opinions can be very helpful in the long run.

While men are likely to tell their significant others they don't need to change anything, women tend to be much more encouraging and supportive of husbands or boyfriends who are considering a cosmetic plastic procedure. As I mentioned in chapter 1, men these days are just as interested in looking better and feeling better about their appearance, although they may not always be as open about it. Having their partners support them makes it easier for them to discuss and pursue the option. According to the American Society of Aesthetic Plastic Surgery (ASAPS), there was a 106 percent increase in the number of men undergoing cosmetic plastic surgery between 1997 and 2012.[17]

It is not uncommon for a man to come in for a procedure after his wife or girlfriend has had a procedure and is extremely happy with her result. Sometimes he comes in at the encouragement of the wife or girlfriend, sometimes it's because he sees how happy she is with her outcomes, and sometimes it is because he wants to turn back the clock alongside his now "younger-looking" wife. I even had a male patient swear his wife encouraged him to have some work done so she could "justify" her ongoing Botox treatments.

According to the American Society of Plastic Surgeons, couples' cosmetic plastic surgery is no longer reserved just for baby boomers.[18] It is starting to become more common for couples to stagger cosmetic plastic procedures, which allows them to be supportive of each other in recovery.

---

17   Megan Willett, "Here's Why There's a 'Huge Boom' in Men Getting Plastic Surgery," Business Insider, March 3, 2014, accessed May 6, 2017, http://www.businessinsider.com/male-plastic-surgery-procedures-2014-2.

18   Anita Patel, "Couples Plastic Surgery by the Decade," American Society of Plastic Surgeons, October 27, 2015, accessed May 6, 2017, https://www.plasticsurgery.org/news/blog/couples-plastic-surgery-by-the-decade.

That is an important piece of advice for recovery from a procedure: if someone is going to be taking care of a spouse or significant other, that person must be involved and invested in what's going on. For instance, if one partner is the primary housekeeper, the other needs to understand it may be up to him or her to pick up the slack while the other partner recovers.

From the patient's perspective, it is also imperative to help spouses and significant others feel comfortable about their decisions to have cosmetic plastic procedures. Patients need to help others understand that even though they are doing the procedure for themselves, they want and need others around them for support. As mentioned earlier, patients can be extremely emotional immediately after having their procedure. They need love, support, and help from their family and friends while recovering.

There are two reasons to get buy-in from others. The first is that patients need proper care as they recover. They need a willing and able family member, friend, or other person to help care for them during the recovery time. The second reason is that since there are no guarantees with cosmetic plastic surgery, outcomes may be seen from a subjective point of view by those who were opposed to the process in the first place. If, for instance, a challenge occurs, healing can take longer if the patient has to deal with an "I told you so" attitude from a nonsupportive family member. Results may even be judged differently: minimal scarring that is acceptable to the patient may be viewed as unacceptable by someone else; a husband may never be "OK" with a scar on his wife if he wasn't on board with her having the procedure. So planning for the surgery before-hand is as important as planning afterward to ensure that everything goes smoothly and you have the best chance of getting the best results.

As a plastic surgeon, I realize it is crucial that I understand the patient's motivation since it is often critical to predicting whether the patient will ultimately be satisfied. For the most part, I have found that women rarely choose to have surgery solely to please their husbands or boyfriends, although I've often wondered if patients tell me they're pursuing plastic surgery for themselves because they think it's the thing to say to me, or they're trying to justify in their own mind why they want it. Too often, people, especially those close to the patient, almost seem to assume there's some ulterior motive for undergoing cosmetic plastic surgery, when in reality, it's usually just because the patient wants to feel better, look better, move better, and be better for others. So there are tremendous differences in the perception of the reason for having cosmetic plastic surgery. For instance, a woman may be having breast implants to look better in a sundress, not because she wants to be the center of attention. She's having the procedure not because she wants to be the center of attention; she does not want to feel "odd" or stand out because her clothes don't seem to fit her properly.

> Too often, people, especially those close to the patient, almost seem to assume there's some ulterior motive for undergoing cosmetic plastic surgery, when in reality, it's usually just because the patient wants to feel better, look better, move better, and be better for others.

Obviously, it is never a good idea to go into a cosmetic plastic procedure with someone else's view of who you are or how you should appear. As I've mentioned, people who undergo cosmetic plastic surgery for someone else or to prove a point are rarely happy with their results. Doing something for yourself and making yourself feel comfortable is far more important than worrying about what others think. Those who hope that plastic surgery will change who they are and how happy they are in their lives are always disappointed, no matter how well the procedure may go and the quality of the end result. While cosmetic plastic surgery can boost your confidence by improving an area of your body that you find dissatisfying, it is not a surgical solution for changing how you perceive others view you. I often think of the young lady I mentioned in the introduction whose husband said, "You're not as beautiful as I need you to be." It must be devastating to hear something like that from your own spouse.

Once I have noted the patients' motivations for plastic surgery, I let them know there are two parts to the surgery process: pre- and postsurgical. The more the patient puts into the presurgical aspect, the easier the process and the postsurgical process will be. That's easier to do when expectations are discussed and understood in advance. Patients who understand that a cosmetic plastic surgery procedure is not being done *to* them but *with* their involvement tend to have a much smoother, more streamlined experience. Patients need to engage in the process with the surgeon as opposed to trying to alter the process because of others' opinions and internet information. We're all on the same team, and we all have the same goal, which is successfully getting you, the patient, safely through the process with the best possible results. That's how we all win.

The good news is that patients' partners who were hesitant at the outset of a procedure come in later to tell us that their significant other looks happier and more refreshed. "She was beautiful before," they often tell us, "but I can definitely see a difference. She looks healthier, more relaxed, more rested." The best compliment I heard a husband pay after his wife's procedure was, "I am happy for her and how happy she is now."

When done for the right reasons, cosmetic plastic surgery can have a profoundly positive effect on your life.

"LIFE IS INHERENTLY RISKY. THERE IS ONLY ONE BIG RISK YOU SHOULD AVOID AT ALL COSTS, AND THAT IS THE RISK OF DOING NOTHING."

—DENIS WAITLEY

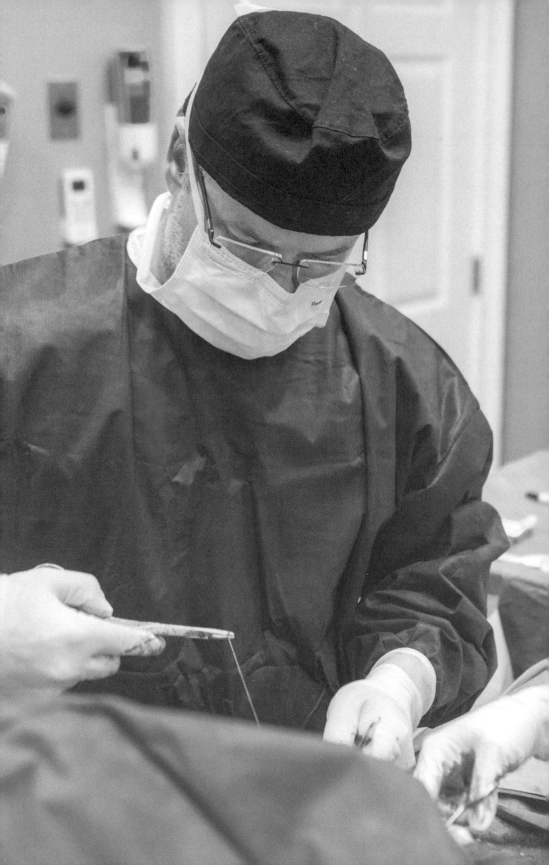

CHAPTER 9

"Google, Aunt Betty, the Florist, and My Chiropractor Said ... "

I'VE BEEN ONLINE, AND I KNOW THAT'S PROBABLY NOT A GOOD THING, BUT I READ ...

T wo weeks after Nora had undergone liposuction, she returned to my office for a postoperative visit. The nurse practitioner checked her treatment areas, removed her dressings, and conducted an overall assessment to determine how Nora was healing. Everything was fine, and she was scheduled for a second postoperative visit two weeks later to see me. In that second visit, I greeted her by jokingly asking, "Are we still friends?" Plastic surgery can be painful, and I know that can sometimes play into a patient's initial reaction following a procedure.

Few people come out of anesthesia with the initial thought that the elective procedure they just underwent was a good idea.

Nora laughed, and I asked if she had any questions, to which she replied, "Yes, I have a few. I went online and googled this procedure and found a lot of pretty scary information. Maybe I shouldn't have looked, but now I'm wondering—does this wound look like it's infected?" She pointed to the area where the procedure had been performed. Although she still had some swelling and bruising, there was no infection, and the tissue was healing as it should, so I assured her everything was fine.

In an age when information is available 24/7, at a person's fingertips, interactions like the one I had with Nora are very common. Everyone has access to the internet, which is loaded with information—some of it misinformation. Or they have a family member or friend who is not in the medical field but who has endless recommendations about surgical management. Often that advice comes from that person's individual experience as a patient under another medical provider—a family physician, a surgical procedure, or even an emergency room visit. News and information today isn't about quality; it's about quantity. It doesn't matter whether it's accurate or useful; it's only about

> Everyone has access to the internet, which is loaded with information—some of it misinformation.

making "noise." Medical circles aren't immune. Just look at what happened early in the COVID-19 pandemic, when the internet was filled with misinformation early on simply because of a lack of information. I like to joke that social media platforms are full of expert virologists these days, many of whom have no formal education or experience in the medical field but have keyboards and Facebook accounts.

The endless desire to help others by giving advice based on something read online or from their own experience is a phenomenon I call the Aunt-Betty-Said syndrome. For patients who have undergone cosmetic plastic surgery, there can be a lot of misunderstanding about recovery, and advice from "Aunt Betty," and the internet, and even physicians from other specialties, can exacerbate the situation. Just as no one else can define beauty for you, *no one else should be giving you advice about how to care for the site of your procedure during recovery except the surgeon who operated on you or an equally trained specialist in the same field.*

Unfortunately, when a perceived challenge arises, instead of consulting the surgeon who performed the procedure, patients sometimes read enough online or consult enough friends or family members that they come to believe their situation to be dire. I'm always amazed at how quickly people who have placed their trust in a plastic surgeon will turn for answers to someone outside the realm of plastic surgery when they think something is not going as it should with their recovery. That trust patients have in their plastic surgeon can be very fragile in some instances, a problem compounded by the internet. There is an insane amount of black box medical information that people can read online, but much of it was not written by a qualified healthcare provider. More importantly, I can't overemphasize the point that no two cases, surgeries, clinical scenarios, or patients are the exact same, and therefore their processes will vary greatly.

Patients seem to want only answers that coincide with what they want to hear. It's almost as if society has become a small child who keeps on asking a question after being told no. Some patients will keep asking until they get a yes, until they're told something they want to hear. They may come back to my office and be told that their wound is healing normally, only to then go to the emergency room or wound care center, where they will be told the wound is infected. But those facilities don't get paid unless there is a diagnosis or a "problem."

When it comes to recovery, I tell patients, "I can't make your wound heal more quickly, but no one cares more about your outcomes than I do. I want you to be happy with your results. I want to see your smiling face when you come back to my office for progress visits." And at my practice, we're willing to do whatever it takes to achieve that goal. I annually invest a lot in training, staff development, modern technology, advertising—everything needed to build a thriving practice. But in the end, my patients' outcomes are what ultimately dictate the success of this business. In spite of what seems to be skepticism on the part of some patients and many patients' family members, my only ulterior motive is to make patients happy. That's what determines my success. Patient happiness is what motivates us— *customer (patient) satisfaction is, simply put, the lifeline of our business.*

But when patients see their situation as dire, they often head over to the local emergency room. There, the "ER wound surgeon" gives them advice that is outside his or her specialty, which then leads to a difficult relationship between the patient and the plastic surgeon who performed the procedure.

> Patient happiness is what motivates us—*customer (patient) satisfaction is, simply put, the lifeline of our business.*

By the way, there is no such thing as an "ER wound surgeon." Yet patients sometimes claim that is who prescribed an antibiotic, pain medication, or wound treatment that is inconsistent with the plastic surgeon's instructions.

Fear of an infection is the main reason some patients head to the ER postsurgery, seeking antibiotics. To reiterate: The payment or reimbursement for the hospital emergency room as well as wound care centers is based on a diagnosis and the complexity of that diagnosis. ER staff members get paid to take care of a problem, but first they have to identify one. In fact, studies have found that patient-satisfaction surveys are an ill-defined measure of true quality delivered by a practice, since their results are often based on whether the patients were denied an antibiotic, pain medication, or other service that they actually didn't need. So even when no infection is present, out of a desire to be helpful and authoritative—and unfortunately, in some instances, to generate revenue or perhaps to comply with a patient-satisfaction mandate—an ER physician will conduct tests or make diagnoses that are not accurate and that instill even more anxiety in the patient.

For the same reason, patients sometimes turn to their primary care physicians for wound treatment following plastic surgery. Admittedly, primary care physicians are knowledgeable about many areas of medicine. Their role is to help patients with routine care and initial workups before identifying which specialists may offer more specialized care. But it is a bad idea for physicians or surgeons to give advice to patients outside the realm of their expertise. If you're truly unhappy, get with your surgeon who performed the procedure and have an honest discussion with them regarding your concerns, but then be willing to listen to their answers and plan with an open mind.

If you're truly unhappy, get with your surgeon who performed the procedure and have an honest discussion with them regarding your concerns, but then be willing to listen to their answers and plan with an open mind.

Having performed tens of thousands of cosmetic plastic procedures, I am confident in addressing the wound needs of my patients, or of any patient who has undergone a cosmetic plastic procedure. That is part of my area of specialty. However, there are various approaches and theories about wound care that are based on the training and experience of the attending physician. My approach is based on my experience and training, and it may be different from another surgeon's approach. In short, there is no absolutely perfect way to manage any particular wound. That can be confusing and frustrating for patients to understand, especially when combined with the fact that wounds that open often appear to get worse before they get better, a part of the protective process of wound healing known as demarcating. When they go back to their surgeon for a review of the healing process and are told that it's normal, they don't necessarily know that the wound may look worse than it does on the day of the checkup before it finally starts getting better. Unfortunately, patients perceive this worsening of symptoms as indicative of a more serious underlying problem and often feel the surgeon is not addressing the issue. It's not that the surgeon doesn't care; it's that there's nothing more that can be done at that point.

While I have been double board certified—by the American Board of Plastic Surgery and the American Board of Surgery—and I delivered a number of babies in medical school, I would not want a patient to call on me to deliver a baby today. Obstetrics are outside my specialty, and delivering babies is not something I do every day. Similarly, even though I worked on a number of cardiothoracic cases as a resident, I'm not a cardiac surgeon, so I would not give advice on recovering from a heart procedure. In fact, women undergoing breast reconstruction often ask me questions about managing their cancer. I tell them those questions must be directed to their oncologists.

So even though there are countless photos and stories online depicting instances of challenges arising following a procedure, those postings do not usually represent the norm. Let's face it: online postings are often done by people who are upset about an experience or a challenge they have had. One person's bad experience does not translate to everyone's bad experience—or *your* bad experience. I think it is safe to say, in general, a patient doesn't want to go to a surgeon who has only done the procedure they want one time, or has never done it, but would rather go to a surgeon who has experience with the procedure. So why would a patient want to listen to someone who may only have had a similar procedure once or who only heard about their friends' experiences with the surgery? It's not a good idea, yet patients do it all the time via social media or the internet.

That's why open lines of communication between patient and surgeon are so important. That preoperative rapport is crucial to a successful outcome, especially if problems or wound-healing challenges arise. The more open the dialogue you have with your surgeon in advance, the more confident you can be of the overall process, the less skepticism you may experience, and the easier the whole process will be.

As I mentioned previously, plastic surgery often involves closing tissue that is under tension or has had its blood supply altered due to the elevation of the tissue necessary to perform the procedure. That can be completely different from other types of surgical wounds. With a cosmetic plastic surgery procedure, tissue is often moved and pulled together to create the desired outcome. Therefore, it is not uncommon for a small area along the incision site to open during the healing process. As does the fear of infection, an open suture can also cause panic among some patients, sending them to the internet for answers, calling Aunt Betty for advice, or heading off to the emergency room thinking the site can be sutured back together.

But resuturing the site is often not the best way to deal with open sutures following cosmetic plastic surgery. Wound tissue is very friable (easily damaged) in the first six weeks after surgery. Friable tension may or may not hold sutures well. If the sutures open, whether because of tension or blood flow or bacteria, we usually let them heal by what is known as "secondary intention," which means allowing the tissue to come together on its own as opposed to being sutured together. Wounds that are wide but not deep usually require only washing, maybe an antibiotic cream, and a new dressing. Occasionally, a suture or two can be used to relieve tension from the healing suture line as a way of keeping the wound from opening further or to protect an underlying implant from exposure. Currently, we often suggest using a well-known wound and burn cream known as Silvadene, soap (baby shampoo is great), and water.

Here is what can happen in the emergency room. The attending physician or surgeon will test the wound and find that it contains bacteria. Everyone has bacteria on their skin, no matter how well the skin is cleaned or prepped before an incision. These bacteria are *colonized*, which means they are at the site helping to fight off the bad bacteria that cause infection. If a wound opens slightly, a test by the ER doctor may show the presence of bacteria, but if the patient does not have a high fever, redness around the wound, or signs of cellulitis (a deeper bacterial infection), antibiotics may not be needed.

In an effort to raise awareness about challenges, risk factors associated with any procedure should always be part of the presurgical consultation. If patients are likely to develop an infection because of a known health condition, their lifestyle, or other factors, that should be discussed in the consultation prior to the surgery. Again, human tissue is dynamic, and there are no guarantees with plastic surgery. But the surgeon's expertise should allow him or her to gauge acceptable parameters associated with the risks.

Healing following a plastic surgery procedure is so misunderstood that, for some patients, it comes with the notion that the surgeon is not owning up to problems, that he or she is downplaying them. However, just as any other medical providers do, plastic surgeons want their patients to have good outcomes. We want people to be happy with their results! Again, no one wants you to heal faster and better than I, the surgeon who performed the procedure. Making you happy is my only ulterior motive.

> Healing following a plastic surgery procedure is so misunderstood that, for some patients, it comes with the notion that the surgeon is not owning up to problems, that he or she is downplaying them.

Contrary to what online resources or other people may suggest, follow-up treatment may not need to be aggressive, and it need not involve the cost of an emergency room visit. Since plastic surgery is rarely reimbursed by medical insurance, pursuing treatment outside the plastic surgeon's plan of care will incur additional, unnecessary costs. That means an emergency room visit for an issue related to cosmetic plastic surgery will often be denied coverage by the insurance company. If it turns out that a perceived infection was simply a normal part of the healing process, the patient may incur a huge bill for something that could have been taken care of in the plastic surgeon's office.

So the plastic surgeon who performed the procedure should be the healthcare provider consulted whenever there is a challenge—real or perceived—following a plastic surgery procedure. That goes back to the relationship I discussed in chapters 5 and 6. It is best to work with the plastic surgeon from the initial consult through the recovery stage. If there is any indication at the initial consult that you feel uneasy or may not be able to openly communicate with the surgeon, you need to reevaluate before proceeding. Surgery is a tough process to maneuver through without complicating it further by having underlying tension. Communication is crucial to a successful plastic surgery experience.

Sometimes, of course, that is not feasible. There are times when the patient is not comfortable continuing the relationship with the surgeon after the procedure. When that occurs, the patient should still seek out a physician or surgeon who specializes in the type of procedure that was performed. Going to the primary care doctor and having him or her become the sole caregiver postoperatively just doesn't make sense. Worse, it can complicate the issue and make the patient more anxious and unsure, further straining the initial surgeon–patient relationship. I've actually had patients tell me that their doctor or nurse friend advised them to do something different from what I had instructed. When I ask, "What kind of doctor?" I'm told he or she is a psychiatrist. Or when I ask, "What kind of nurse?" I'm told that he or she is a pediatric nurse. There's a definitive line between treatment recommendations based on hard-core medical knowledge and treatment recommendations from a friend—even a friend with some level of medical knowledge—who is trying to be supportive.

If patients tell me they are unhappy with the care they receive from me, I understand, but I want to make sure they find someone who can give them the right guidance and instruction so that their procedure turns out well in the long run. Conversely, as I mentioned earlier, when patients come to me from another provider, I prefer to quell the drama and move forward with care to help them get the best outcome possible. I refuse to degrade or insult other surgeons or their work. I also don't critique or give negative feedback to a patient who's already anxious. Since I wasn't in on the initial surgery, the best course of action I can take is to offer my recommendation for moving forward.

At times, patients perceive delays in healing where there are none because the plastic surgeon did not spend enough time educating the patient in advance of the procedure. Remember that plastic surgeons spend nearly ten years in training beyond high school, followed by six to seven years of surgical training, during which they perform not only surgery but also preoperative and postoperative management. So their knowledge of what can happen, normally happens, and rarely happens is far greater than that of a nonmedical professional who has undergone plastic surgery or any medical professional who has not performed such procedures. That's why it is crucial to choose someone you trust, someone with the right qualifications and experience and who you believe has your best interests at heart. Using Google as an educational source can be enlightening, but it is not authoritative. In fact, I had to laugh at the saying I once saw on a patient's coffee cup: "My medical experience trumps your Google search."

There are a number of ways to ensure you're making a good choice in plastic surgery providers. Look for these best practices to ensure information is communicated to you and that you have a good experience overall.

A good first encounter. Your impression of a plastic surgery provider should begin with the first call you make to the office to set up an initial appointment. Is the office staff member on the other end of the phone friendly? Knowledgeable? Compassionate? Understanding? Even if that person is only setting up an appointment for you, he or she should be able to make you feel comfortable from the first hello and be able to answer some of the initial questions that arise.

First-person experience. In many plastic surgery offices, staff members have actually undergone a cosmetic plastic procedure themselves, so they have firsthand knowledge of the process. When they share their experience, they can help alleviate concerns and put patients at ease. Prospective surgery patients should also ask the surgeon's staff members if they would recommend the surgeon to their family or friends, and whether any of their family or friends subsequently came in for treatment.

Tenure counts. How long has the surgeon's staff been working with him or her? Long-term staff understand how a physician's practice works, which can add to a patient's sense of comfort and a better understanding of how the process works.

An ability to relate. Having staff members who can relate to patients' concerns also helps with communication throughout the process. For instance, at my practice, we have a nurse practitioner and a physician's assistant who are both around the same age and have life experiences that are similar to those of a good portion of our patients. They are generally the first to meet with patients one on one to explain the procedures and give them pre-op information. It's important for patients to know, early on, who the primary point of contact will be throughout the process and to build rapport with that person to help them feel more comfortable.

Part of the pre-op information may include before-and-after photos of other patients' procedures to help new and potential patients get a visual idea of outcomes. In some cases, potential or new patients may even be put in touch with past or current patients to learn about their experiences. You should remember, however, the experiences of other patients are only *examples* of what other people experience and not necessarily what you will experience too.

After meeting with assisting providers, patients should then meet with the surgeon who will perform their procedure. That is when the surgeon has the opportunity to answer any additional questions and help patients make a final decision about which procedure might be best for their situation. That is when to discuss goals and potential outcomes. (Do you want to wear a bikini again, or fit into a certain dress size, or look better for a wedding or reunion?) Understanding a patient's expectations, as I've mentioned, can help alleviate misunderstandings over the long term. The consultation with the surgeon should be followed by an examination to determine whether the desired results can be achieved in the area that is to be treated.

Clarification of costs. Once the examination is completed, costs should be discussed. In most offices, that discussion takes place with the office manager or other financial staff member. The discussion should go over each line item to ensure all questions about costs are clarified. Meeting with a range of staff up front is one of the best ways to help patients feel more comfortable with the process, from start to finish. Revision costs should also be discussed. It's good to know up front what potential revisions could occur along with any potential costs involved.

Clearly written and explained pre-op instructions. There are a number of special instructions that should be explained prior to the procedure. Patients should be required to sign a consent form after reading them and asking questions to clarify anything that is not understood.

These instructions include what is typically required by most surgeries: patients must stop taking certain medications (primarily blood thinners), they are not allowed to eat or drink after a certain time, they must remove all jewelry, and they must arrange to have a ride home. Specifically, for plastic surgery, there are additional instructions including removing all nail polish, showering with a special scrub, drinking plenty of water, taking specific supplements, and stopping smoking.

As with other surgeries, prior to plastic surgery, patients need to stay active and increase their protein intake. The last thing a patient should do right before plastic surgery is try to lose a lot of weight; a body in starvation mode breaks down protein, which is a major component of wound healing. Surgery, in general, causes a stress response in the body. It metabolizes, or breaks down, protein to do the healing. If you have depleted your protein stores by fasting or dieting, your wound healing may be impacted. It is better to be carrying a few extra pounds and be in a good nutritional state when having plastic surgery rather than to try to quickly lose some weight with a crash diet. That goes for tummy tucks as well—even with a little bit of additional weight, you can still have good outcomes.

Ideally, cosmetic plastic surgery is for patients who are within 10 percent of their ideal weight. Obese patients should get to a healthier body weight before having a procedure.

Postsurgery contacts. A patient's discharge paperwork should contain contact information, including a phone number that can be used outside office hours. Usually, the contact is the original main contact assigned to the case, which helps avoid confusion and frustration for the patient. Technology today also allows for patients to send photos if they have questions during recovery. These can help determine whether patients should be seen earlier than their next scheduled visit, or whether sufficient care instructions and attention to their concerns can be given over the phone. Offering that availability postsurgery is a lifeline that can help patients feel more comfortable with the procedure.

Go with your gut feeling. Ultimately, go with your gut feeling, since instincts are rarely wrong. If you are comfortable with a person, procedure, or place, then go with it. Equally, if you're uncomfortable, then that is not the right person, procedure, or place for you.

The best way to quell concerns about plastic surgery is to forgo the internet and Aunt Betty for advice—none of them can define beauty for you, and none of them can give you the best advice about plastic surgery. The internet should not be used as a medical diagnostic and management tool. Nor should the experience of others be used by patients to gauge their own experience. At my practice, I tell patients to come in every other day if that's what it takes to really feel assured. Our goal, again, is a happy outcome.

The best information about plastic surgery comes from professionally conducted studies and the data resulting from them. Reviews of medical studies are very useful but need to be understood in terms of their applicability, the source, and the verification protocol.

When studies and other data do not provide answers, people often turn to online reviews to determine whether to engage a provider. A word of caution: Anyone with a keyboard can type up a blog that has no medical credentials and is not vetted for accuracy. It is all too easy to believe a negative review by someone who claims to have had a bad experience with a provider. Rarely are the reviewers looking at the material from an educational perspective. Usually, they are not discussing the technicalities of the procedure; more often than not, they are just venting. There is rarely, if ever, any explanation of how or why challenges arose.

Review platforms cater to the customer and reviewer. Disgruntled former employees, competitors—anyone—can go online and leave a review; there is no vetting to ensure the persons leaving the comment actually had the experience they are describing. The sites are not designed to aid the business or truly educate the consumer.

I speak from experience about bad reviews. A few years back, a former patient posted a bad review because she was upset about her wound healing. What she failed to mention, however, was that I had insisted that she quit smoking, and she did not. She continued to smoke after her procedure. Smoking can have a detrimental effect on healing, reducing circulation to the skin and impeding new tissue growth. Patches should also be avoided when having plastic surgery because they have nicotine in them. Even secondhand smoke can cause problems with plastic surgery.

In recognition of the need for a better, more accurate online review process, I've developed a software review platform for physicians, veterinarians, chiropractors, and others. Known as Loopit, and found at goloopit.com, the platform validates patients before allowing them to leave a review. Only patients who have set up an appointment with a doctor or have had a procedure can leave a review. The platform allows for physicians and health/wellness providers and businesses to respond to reviews, helping to clarify misunderstandings or allowing them to weigh in with additional details that may not have been revealed in the patient's review.

Visit goloopit.com.

The platform gives patients a chance to see how providers handle negative reviews, because no provider can guarantee everything will go exactly right 100 percent of the time. It also allows for posting medical articles to give providers a chance to show, for instance, that some level of scarring occurs in every procedure. In addition, this program elicits useful, informative reviews using a formatted template technique, which alleviates the emotional rants that are so common on most review platforms today. Such postings, along with the interaction, can help educate the consumer and bring a better understanding than, say, a Google search.

As a patient, your role is to ensure that what you want aligns with what you are being told. Then, if you choose to move forward, you must realize that you are committing to a process and you must be fair to that process. That's what healing and recovery is about. If you undergo a surgical procedure with the understanding that it will take three months for your incision scar to begin to show signs of improvement, then that's your role as a patient: to commit to that timeline and see it through. If you need a second opinion to feel comfortable, be sure that second opinion is from a valid source, not your friend, your neighbor, or your psychiatrist. Even though the latter is a doctor, he or she is not qualified to diagnose a healing plastic surgery wound.

> As a patient, your role is to ensure that what you want aligns with what you are being told.

Aunt Betty, a great lady, may have lots of world experience, but even if she is in the medical field, the bottom line is simple: unless she's a plastic surgeon who regularly performs the type of procedure you had done, she's not qualified to give you advice about how your wound is healing. Why would you listen to somebody who has limited or no experience but is telling you what you want to hear, as opposed to a person with experience who only wants to see you have a great outcome?

It is great to have a sympathetic friend or family member in your corner. In fact, such support is crucial to a good postoperative recovery. But would you let a friend or family member perform plastic surgery on you? No. Then you should not be taking their advice about wound healing after a plastic surgery procedure. An emergency room doctor who tells you what you need to have done but doesn't have the credentials to do the procedure himself or herself is not giving you the best medical advice for your situation.

Just as you can't let others advise you over wound healing, you can't let them define beauty for you. Remember that beauty is subjective: what seems beautiful to someone else—Aunt Betty, your florist, Google, or otherwise—may not make you feel beautiful.

"PEOPLE WILL STARE.
MAKE IT WORTH
THEIR WHILE."

—HARRY WINSTON

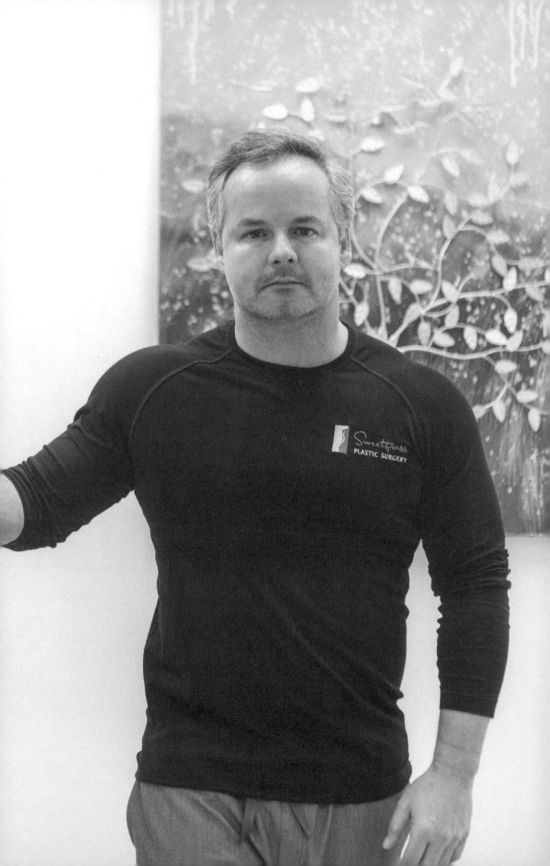

CHAPTER 10

"Not Gonna Happen to Me"

WHY IS THIS HAPPENING? DO YOU NEED TO STITCH IT SHUT AGAIN?

Beth was in her midforties when she came in for a breast lift and augmentation. A mother of two, she had decided to "get her body back" after childbirth had left her breasts asymmetrical and with less mass.

During my presurgical consultation with her, I informed Beth that there is always scarring with such procedures. I explained that the degree of scarring varies greatly from patient to patient and is based on the type of procedure, genetics, and how she cared for herself following the surgery. For example, scars that are very red, raised, firm, and can even itch or burn are called immature scars, and they take nine to twelve months to fully mature for most skin types. I explained that wound healing after breast augmentation and a lift can be an issue because the procedure involves pulling the tissue very tightly together over the implant, and it is not uncommon for the incision underneath the breast to open a bit during healing. I explained the other risks involved and the steps she should take if an issue—such as the wound opening—happened during her recovery. I also explained that should the wound open, we would address it later—after the wound had fully healed, since trying to alter it any sooner would basically be like trying to hit a moving target. Scars lighten and flatten dramatically over time. People with very fair skin, blue eyes, or red hair (as was the case with Beth) often deal with very red scars that can take a year to calm down. My goal was to help Beth to really understand the process ahead of time, which is my goal for all my patients. Beth agreed that everything we had talked about was acceptable. She signed the consent forms and soon had the procedures done with no issues during the surgery. "If I can bear children, I'm sure I can make it through plastic surgery just fine," she commented.

Four days after her surgery, Beth called into the office, worried sick that the wound was infected. I had her send in pictures of the wound, which revealed that a small area along the incision had opened. It was not a large area and therefore nothing to really be alarmed about. With a little extra care—keeping the wound clean and applying an antibiotic ointment and a clean dressing—I assured Beth that she would be fine until she returned for her appointment early the following week.

When she arrived at the office for that postoperative visit, she immediately asked me, "Why did my suture open? Do you have to go in and do more work on me now?" I examined the areas of her procedure, including the area that had opened, and it was doing just fine. Beth had followed my over-the-phone instructions—to the letter, it appeared—and she was healing as expected. Everything, including the open area, was continuing to improve and was on track to heal with minimal scarring. I reminded her that once her swelling and edema had subsided and she was fully healed, we would look at the wound again to determine whether the scarring would need additional treatment. If needed at that time, we could remove the scar itself and resuture skin, and then it would heal tremendously.

Beth's experience demonstrates how patients often undergo plastic surgery believing they will have the best outcomes, only to have challenges arise that cause them grief and sleepless nights.

Open wounds are scary to patients. I completely understand that. Obviously, I see them every day, but to most patients, a surgical wound is something new and different. It can be even scarier to family and friends who haven't been through the preoperative discussion with the surgeon. So, of course, many wonder how their wound can possibly heal—yet the wound does heal. All it takes is a little patience.

Again, skin naturally has bacteria that contaminate an open wound. The age-old surgical soap and water is well known as the most effective cleaning agent. Years ago, surgeons used to advise letting a wound dry out or desiccate. Today, it's recommended to keep the wound hydrated, either with a certain cream or a petroleum-based ointment, which have been shown to improve the wound-healing process.

If a wound is open with tissue that needs to be removed (debrided), that condition can be addressed, in part, with wet-to-dry dressing care. That involves dampening a small piece of gauze with a saline solution and laying it on the wound. As it dries, it attaches to the unwanted tissue. When the dressing is removed, it also debrides, or removes, the unwanted tissue. The wound may bleed after the treatment, but that is healthy granulation bleeding. This technique is especially useful for wounds that are deep or that have undermining or tunneling associated with them.

Again, wounds that are open or start to open often get worse before they get better. And that takes days or even weeks. It really depends on the patient's physiology. Unfortunately, as I've mentioned, suturing a wound that has opened is not a solution; tissue that is inflamed and pliable really won't hold sutures. The good news is that scars will mature, and once they've finished healing, there are a number of treatment options available.

An enormous amount of time goes into pre-op discussions of risks, benefits, and alternative therapies, in addition to gaining the consent of patients who acknowledge that they understand and accept the risks. Many or most patients today do some kind of online research, which gives them a different understanding of the procedure from what is being presented to them by the surgeon.

Even after explaining all that is involved in plastic surgery, many patients do not believe that the rules apply to them. They don't understand that the statistics are based on averages culled from a large sampling of people and that they fall within those averages. Being one of the "averages," in essence, makes them normal. Still, they undergo surgery believing they will sail through with no hitches, even when statistics show otherwise. For instance, many people claim they heal quickly, they have high pain tolerance, or they will be back to work a week after a procedure that generally requires more recovery time. Unfortunately, they are not grasping the reality of the situation. Most surgeries do not allow people to get back to their daily lives so quickly. And while they may have healed well when they were younger, twenty years later, their body has likely changed—significantly. Physiologic age versus chronologic age can make a big difference in a person's ability to heal. A sixty-year-old who exercises regularly and eats right may heal better than an out-of-shape forty-year-old who drinks and smokes and has hypertension and diabetes.

Mental health can also play a significant role in healing. Even those who seem to "have it all together" can heal more slowly if they are anxious or are significantly stressed in their personal or profes-sional life. That's because anxiety raises levels of cortisol in the blood-stream, and cortisol blocks the body's inflammatory response (that rush of white blood cells that I discussed in chapter 7). Those white blood cells are needed to help heal the incision. In addition, anxiety or stress causes a release of catecholamines (stress hormones), which can also constrict the flow of blood to the tiny vessels in the skin and at the leading edge of a wound, and that blood flow is vital to good healing. This is the same effect as nicotine. If a wound does not heal primarily, meaning the edges don't mend together but instead spread apart or open up, that wound has to heal secondarily, which basically means tissue fills in over the wound and creates a wider scar that may need to be addressed later.

Yes, there are real risks with any procedure. But if you think about it, avoiding all the risks in life would mean never leaving the house! Where would we be today if the generations before us never took some risks?

Still, to alleviate some concerns, let me share with you some of the most common challenges that can occur with plastic surgery:

- Hematomas, which appear as bruises, occur in 1 to 6 percent of breast augmentation surgeries, and in many face lifts. Hematomas may dissipate on their own; if not, they will need to be drained or evacuated.[19]

- Hypertrophic scarring, which is a raised, red scar, occurs in 2 to 5 percent of patients. These can often be repaired with additional treatment.[20]

---

19   "The 10 Most Common Plastic Surgery Complications," Healthline, accessed May 28, 2017, http://www.healthline.com/health/most-common-plastic-surgery-complications#1.

20   Ibid.

- Cellulitis, a skin infection, occurs in 2 to 4 percent of patients undergoing breast surgeries.[21] Patients can sometimes require antibiotics to get their healing process back on track.

- Nerve damage can occur with plastic surgery and is potentially indicated by tingling and/or numbness.[22]

- Keloids are superaggressive scars that typically form a smooth, hard surface. Although unattractive, they are not harmful. People with darker pigmented skin tend to be more at risk for keloid scars.[23]

> Yes, there are real risks with any procedure. But if you think about it, avoiding all the risks in life would mean never leaving the house!

In spite of a surgeon's in-depth explanation of the common and less common consequences of surgery, some patients have great difficulty in accepting this information. They read and sign the consent forms, and we talk about the physical conditions that are expected to occur in the course of healing after their type of procedure, yet they are still surprised, and sometimes even angry, when they experience the same physical reactions that other patients have.

Even though cosmetic plastic surgery enjoys a low rate of post-operative problems—1.4 percent of cosmetic plastic procedures end in significant challenges—patients tend to believe they could never be

---

21   Ibid.

22   Ibid.

23   "Keloid Scar of Skin," Healthline, accessed July 5, 2017, http://www.healthline.com/health/keloids#overview1.

one of the few who do experience a negative outcome.[24] Again, plastic surgery is not an exact science; that is explained ahead of surgery. Challenges can and do arise, and when they do, as I've said, some patients want to blame the surgeon or staff members or the process itself—thinking something must have gone wrong for the suture to open—instead of accepting that they are simply among the few who have a negative experience. Quite often, patients come to me blaming another doctor for "butchering" them simply because their outcomes were not what they expected. For these patients, even minor problems seem huge.

When it comes to problems, levels of severity vary from *likely outcomes*, meaning common or likely problems (e.g., infections and slow-to-heal wounds), and problems caused by *true malpractice*, which means acting outside what is considered within the realm of normal care.

Too often in the medical profession, patients want to sue for malpractice because their outcomes did not meet their expectations. Unhappy or dissatisfied patients don't equate to malpractice; they simply equate to unhappy patients. But small setbacks, such as sutures opening early during the healing process, are not causes for malpractice lawsuits. Unfortunately, today there are doctors who make a living giving testimonies in court while not actively practicing medicine or performing hands-on surgery from day to day. They usually testify on behalf of patients who are making a claim arising from a complex medical procedure of which they have no expertise or medical knowledge. Plaintiffs' surgeons often sell their opinions for the right price to help bring a suit against colleagues. In addition,

---

24   Wolters Kluwer Health: Lippincott Williams and Wilkins, "'Tummy Tuck' Complications: Study Looks at Rates and Risk Factors," ScienceDaily, news release, October 29, 2015, accessed May 27, 2017, www.sciencedaily.com/releases/2015/10/151029124815.htm.

plaintiffs' lawyers have private online resources—communities of lawyers in their geographic area—that only they can access. They use these to fish for potentially negative information about a doctor, such as his or her past interactions with other lawyers or unhappy patients, that can be used in a suit against the doctor. Without these "secret" resources, lawyers must rely on public records of filed lawsuits. (I have often thought about starting my own website citing the misbehaviors and transgressions of lawyers, although I'm sure that would put me in the crosshairs of one of those private lawyer sites, not to mention I'm sure it is "illegal.")

So while medical malpractice is very real in some cases, in others, it is surreal and frustrating—and the reason a lot of medical professionals leave medicine. A physician can do everything right and still be sued because a patient with no medical knowledge claims a procedure was done improperly or mismanaged postoperatively. The biggest problems seem to occur after a confrontation between the patient and the surgeon, usually because of a level of mistrust that has developed from outside influences on the patient. And ironically, most lawsuits are brought by not only a patient but also a lawyer, neither of who has any medical experience or knowledge, and they are tried in front of juries with no medical experience or background. Despite signing an informed consent agreement, patients still claim they did not know or understand the risks or potential challenges. Plaintiffs' attorneys will often claim that plaintiffs' preoperative awareness of the risks and their signatures on the consent form don't negate the possibility of malpractice. But nowhere on the consent form does it say that problems only occur if the doctor does something wrong. The bottom line is that despite strict adherence to standards, despite a perfectly executed procedure, challenges still arise for a percentage of patients. The surgeon can follow protocol, the patient can adhere to postsurgical directions, and setbacks in healing can still occur. That's because, again, plastic surgery and the healing of body tissue are not an exact science; there are no guarantees, even if everything is followed to the letter. That's what the consent form is trying to convey to the patient.

A lot of the reasons for malpractice suits go back to expectations. When patients suffer a setback, such as a wound opening, it is very real and sometimes very scary for them. They want to know exactly when to expect their wound to heal. They want to know what a scar will look like. Even doing the math—new skin grows on a wound site at the rate of about one millimeter per day—it can only be estimated when a wound may heal. And even knowing roughly how long a wound will take to close is no indicator of how the scar will turn out. Slow-to-heal wounds do not mean the final outcome will be a bad one. Ultimately, expectations and communication are key to any patient-doctor relationship.

Patients also cannot base their expectations on other patients' outcomes. Patients sometimes come in wanting a physical feature (e.g., lips, nose, breasts) to look just like a friend's, but since everyone is unique, what works for one patient may not work for another. Plastic surgery is not a cookie-cutter process. A woman may say she wants the

> Ultimately, expectations and communication are key to any patient-doctor relationship.

same size of breast implants as a friend has, but those implants may not work for her. The same implant on ten different patients will look different on each patient, and their healing outcome will look different as well. Even close family members undergoing the same cosmetic plastic surgery procedure cannot expect the same outcome. Fortunately, today, in my practice, we have technology that can more accurately help predict which breast implant will produce the desired outcome. That, along with experience and training, can help produce surgeries and procedures tailored for you, those that are best suited to your body. Still, the expectation of cosmetic plastic surgery delivering perfection complicates the process even further. For instance, women often expect breast augmentation to make their imperfect breasts perfect. It may improve what they were not endowed with, but it may not make them "perfect."

Patients should never be promised a specific outcome or the best possible result. The best any plastic surgeon can do is predict a possible outcome within reason, based on past procedures, combined with a patient's current health and other factors that are known because of the patient-surgeon relationship.

Preoperative consultations and gaining informed consent can help patients better understand that some setbacks are real; they can and do happen. However, most happen infrequently, and by following postoperative measures, they can often be avoided. By informing patients and gaining their consent in advance of procedures, misunderstandings can often be avoided. Instead of glossing over the information presented prior to surgery, patients must be sure to read the information carefully before signing. They need to ask questions and get a clear understanding of what their procedure entails: What are the anticipated outcomes? What kind of timeline for recovery can they realistically expect? Plastic surgery is surgery, after all, and no one wants surprises on the road ahead. As a patient, if you feel the surgeon is not answering your questions or you do not have a clear understanding of what the surgery and postoperative recovery period entails, the time to walk away is before you make the payment, before you allow someone you do not trust to work on you. Walking away from a situation you do not fully trust is in the best interest of everyone.

Even though plastic surgery continues to evolve, as do all medical fields, it still seems to generate a lot of bad press. Breast implants may be the best example of the bad press plastic surgery has had to overcome. Today's breast implants are made of a cohesive silicone gel formula. However, in the 1990s, breast implants contained a saline liquid gel, and a national television news show found five women who had connective tissue disease, which they contracted within a year or two of having a breast augmentation. Connective tissue disease is an autoimmune disease that causes a range of symptoms and affects various areas of the body. The silicone implants were faulted as the cause of the women's disease, so they were taken off the US market for cosmetic plastic use, although they were still used worldwide and were used in the United States for reconstruction. Over time, studies found no correlation between the saline gel and connective tissue disease. Of the estimated two million women who had implants then, five had connective tissue disease, which is a disease that can affect women in their thirties—the ages of the women the news show chose to interview. The largest maker of the implants back then bowed out of the market in the wake of the controversy.

Potentially complicating matters today is that many other types of providers are beginning to offer cosmetic plastic procedures as part of their practices. With reimbursement from medical insurance declining so dramatically, family doctors and ob-gyns are starting to offer liposuction, and oral surgeons and ear, nose, and throat specialists (ENTs) are starting to do facial procedures. They are all trying to tap into what is a cash-for-service industry. Ironically, in most states, almost anyone can get a license to practice medicine and perform surgery, and there are few guidelines for someone in private practice. It takes accreditation by a credentials committee to offer plastic surgery services in a hospital setting. That credentialing, by the American

Board of Plastic Surgery and the American Board of Medical Specialists, is something patients should always look for in a provider.

Certainly, bad things can and do happen in medicine and surgery. Where fault can become a factor is when the surgeon does not take proper care of the patient after the surgery, or the surgeon does not respond to the patient's issues or complaints within what's known as "the standard of care." Essentially, that means the surgeon must comply with the same range of treatments employed by other surgeons in the same profession.

Having a good relationship up front can help overcome any unforeseen challenges. The more the patient knows and understands ahead of time, the easier it is to believe the surgeon when an unforeseen challenge occurs. Without that level of trust, anything the surgeon says is going to sound suspicious or misleading.

Of course, many patients have the credo that they can't live their life in fear. They understand there are no guarantees. They want plastic surgery, they are going to have a procedure done, and they willingly accept the risks involved. They understand that setbacks can arise, and they deal with them if and when they happen. It is the mindset that a setback will never happen—when clearly the risks exist—that leads to problems down the road.

Some people also accept that while they want a plastic surgery procedure, they may have doubts afterward that their decision was a good one. On occasion, while procedures are intended to improve an area, patients may decide after having the procedure that their choice of procedure might not have been the best fit. The outcomes may not match their expectations, but even if the end result is a little less than expected, for the most part, they are still happy they chose to have a procedure done. They like the way they look, their clothes fit better, they feel better wearing a swimsuit or shorts. In fact, occasionally, I am more bothered by an outcome than a patient is. Naomi, for instance, had a scar after her tummy tuck that could have been improved with a minor procedure. But when I asked her if she would like to talk about what we could do to make it look better, she simply replied, "Honestly, it doesn't bother me at all."

Unlike Naomi, some patients will want improvements for the smallest scar, measurable only in millimeters. When a scar is barely noticeable, the amount of improvement a patient will experience should be weighed into whether the procedure is worth the time and expense of undertaking it. If the patients are not happy with a scar that is a millimeter or two wide, they probably will never be happy with any result. That, again, is when other factors may very well be in play: Do these patients have a sense of their own internal beauty, or is someone else defining beauty for them? Making sure a patient's perceived and expected outcome is in line with their probable outcome is absolutely crucial. I believe it is the responsibility of both the patient and the surgeon to ensure this happens prior to any procedure.

There is risk and reward for everything in life, whether it is business or medicine or taking up a hobby. Is what you're trying to achieve worth the risks involved? While most risks are small, they are real. And once you decide to go through with a plastic surgery procedure, the best way to approach it is to go into it with an open mind, accepting that something unwelcome may happen. If it does, you must work through it with your surgeon. Be prepared for the chance that a challenge may occur, and then be glad when everything goes smoothly.

"ALL OUR DREAMS CAN COME TRUE IF WE HAVE THE COURAGE TO PURSUE THEM."

—WALT DISNEY

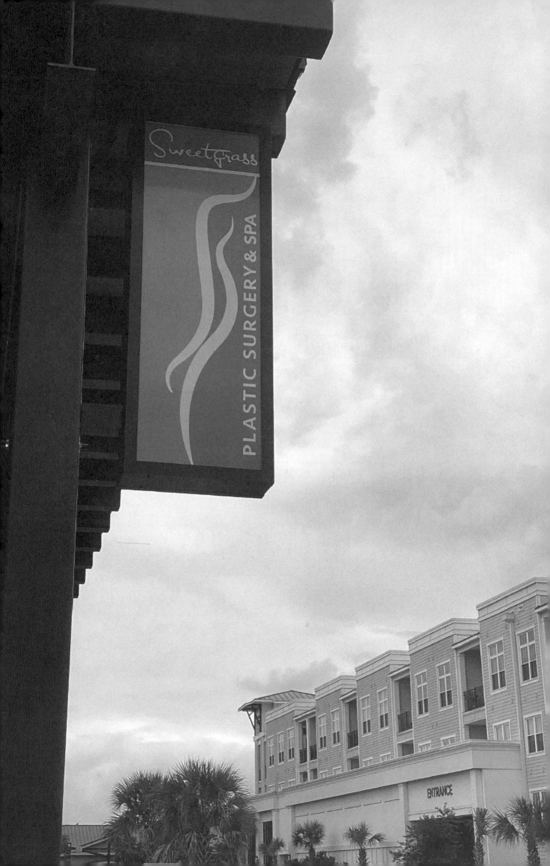

CHAPTER 11

The Evolution of Cosmetic Plastic Surgery and Its Exciting Future

The pursuit of beauty is not something new. People have always been concerned about their appearances. While modern technologies—social media and apps and smartphones—have definitely popularized the concern about appearance, it's something that's always been present.

In fact, plastic surgery dates back 3,000 to 3,500 years, with people looking for ways to improve appearance or fix injuries. Documents dating back to 2500 BC detail a procedure that may be the first record of how to fix a broken nose. Plastic surgery really began to evolve around 800 BC in India, with people undergoing all kinds of procedures, ranging from replacing soft-tissue defects to skin grafts to correct injuries or trauma. Records began being kept of the various treatments, and soon procedures were being done in Italy and then throughout Europe and into Britain.

Fast forward to the 1700s and there were more craniofacial surgeries being done, including surgeries to correct cleft lip and palate defects. The results obviously weren't great by today's comparison, but back then, there was really no point of reference, and people were willing to try unproven things in an effort to look better. There was also no anesthesia back then (anesthesia didn't show up until the mid-1800s), yet they were willing to undergo tremendous pain and risk to improve their appearance because it mattered, even at that point. It really amazes me and makes me cringe a little to think about how they might have been doing some of the bone grafts and tissue transfers back then. I can't imagine how those were being done successfully. Today, we have so much more at our disposal to really make a difference in the results and in the outcome.

"Plastic surgery" comes from the word *plastikē*, which is the art of modeling a malleable material, such as tissue. The term first appeared in 1839, long before the actual development of the material made from petroleum that we know as plastic. Much of plastic surgery's evolution and growth has been dependent on other events such as world wars, trauma, technology, the evolution of anesthesia, and other factors.

> "Plastic surgery" comes from the word *plastikē*, which is the art of modeling a malleable material, such as tissue.

In 1895, the first breast augmentation was performed to correct asymmetry and involved transplanting tissue from the patient's back. Then, the First World War really became the breeding grounds for reconstruction. Unfortunately, the trauma that is a result of war necessitated treatment options. During this time, Dr. Harold Gillies chronicled his work on injured servicemen in his book *Plastic Surgery of the Face*.[25] In the early 1900s, Dr. Vilray Blair developed some innovative skin-grafting techniques and was instrumental in establishing several plastic surgery training facilities at universities and military training operations.[26] With each subsequent war, further advancements in medical care improved, especially in plastic and reconstructive surgery for tissue injuries and soft-tissue reconstruction.

Plastic surgery is a surgical specialty that refers to restoration, reconstruction, or alterations to the human body in one form or another. There are two areas of plastic surgery: reconstruction and cosmetic or aesthetic. Plastic surgery has evolved as a result of both types of surgeries. Doctors who become cosmetic plastic surgeons often start out as reconstructive surgeons. In that capacity, they first learn techniques and how to address complex problems. Having that foundational understanding of the principles of reconstruction is how a plastic surgeon transitions to cosmetic plastic surgery. Those same principles that apply to the reconstruction aspect are what allow us to improve form and appearance through cosmetic surgery. Plastic surgery is probably the only true specialty where we still operate on every part of the body and almost every age range, male or female. We can reconstruct almost any area of the body following cancer surgery, and there are also high areas of specialization, including hand and facial trauma. Then there is microsurgery, which involves moving tissue from one place on the body to another using microscopes.

---

25   Christopher Klein, "Innovative Cosmetic Surgery Restored WWI Vets' Ravaged Faces—And Lives," History.com, October 26, 2018. Accessed February 1, 2020, https://www.history.com/news/world-war-i-plastic-surgery-innovations-gillies.

26   Faisal Ameer, Arun Kumar Singh, and Sandeep Kumar, "Evolution of instruments for harvest of the skin grafts," *Indian Journal of Plastic Surgery*, vol. 46, no. 1(January-April 2013): 28–35. doi: 10.4103/0970-0358.113704.

Reconstruction is generally not solely an elective procedure; it's usually something that needs to be done to improve or restore function and form. Within reconstruction are other subareas, such as facial and bone surgery and microsurgery, which is often used following cancer treatment. Cosmetic plastic surgery is usually elective and is generally chosen to improve appearance, not so much function. Interestingly, that's the defining factor for insurance companies to determine whether a procedure is covered or not—they look at whether it is a reconstruction or cosmetic procedure.

Today, cosmetic plastic surgery is still primarily a female-driven industry. Although it's not understood why, fewer minorities undergo cosmetic plastic surgery. Still, there's been a huge increase in the number of nonsurgical procedures being performed every year: injectables, Botox, fillers, hair removal, lasering, and so on. In 2019, more than eighteen million cosmetic surgical procedures and cosmetic minimally invasive procedures were performed along with another nearly six million reconstructive procedures.[27]

That's a huge number, and it's growing pretty consistently year after year, with social media, advertising, technology really contributing to its explosion.

So the future of plastic surgery is about addressing three things: psychological components, education, and developments in technology and techniques (the basic sciences).

---

27   "Plastic Surgery Report," 2019, American Society of Plastic Surgeons, accessed February 24, 2021, https://www.plasticsurgery.org/documents/News/Statistics/2019/plastic-surgery-statistics-full-report-2019.pdf.

Psychological Components

The expansion of cosmetic plastic surgery has led to an increase in body dysmorphic disorder, which is present in about 2 percent of the general population but is present in an estimated 15 to 20 percent of people who seek out cosmetic plastic surgery. Technology has compounded the problem: a phenomenon titled "Snapchat dysmorphia" describes people who want plastic surgery to make themselves appear as they do when using the app's photo editing filters.[28] In response to the problem, Instagram opted to ban its augmented reality filters.[29] It's an interesting question for plastic surgeons: When someone has body dysmorphia, what do we do? Do we go ahead with the procedure or turn them away? With the latter, they're not going to just go home and forget about it; they're going to seek out alternatives, perhaps higher-risk, more dangerous alternatives—in garages or in less-reputable parts of the world with someone with no experience or training. So in some ways, turning them away is worse than trying to make them happy.

Again, as surgeons, it's really up to us to explore with the patient the reasons they want to have a procedure. What are their goals? During a consult, I try to discover whether someone has a real desire or is just obsessing over something. Again, that's why we have counseling in my practice, and we encourage discussion.

---

28 "A new reality for beauty standards: How selfies and filters affect body image," *Boston Medical Center*, news release, August 2, 2018, accessed February 1, 2020, https://www.sciencedaily.com/releases/2018/08/180802141601.htm.

29 "Instagram bans 'cosmetic surgery' filters," *BBC News*, October 23, 2019, accessed February 1, 2020, https://www.bbc.com/news/business-50152053.

Education

In the past, we plastic surgeons haven't done enough to educate patients and the public. We haven't acknowledged or embraced the psychological complexities that go with plastic surgery. That's something we need to do more of going forward. We need to recognize that there's been a lack of education about what we do, and we need to get better at communicating and educating people.

Today, patients are already somewhat savvier about procedures and options available to them. Because of the internet, they have a lot of information at their fingertips. But it's not always accurate information, nor is it right for their situation, and they don't necessarily understand all that they're reading. It's that whole "having a little knowledge is a dangerous thing" situation, which is something that previous generations of surgeons and doctors in general never faced. Thirty years ago, a doctor would prescribe a medication, and the patient would take it. Now, the patient often says, "Well, I googled that" or "I chatted with someone on the internet who said … " Social media has connected society in such a way that the flow of information is much greater, but it's really difficult to know what the truth is anymore.

In order for plastic surgery to be successful and for patients to be happy, we professionals have to acknowledge our roles in educating patients and helping them sift through the information. If we don't do that, then patients are left to sort through everything that's on the internet, which, again, is not always accurate or right for them.

Still, I do recommend that people considering plastic surgery collect as much data as they can but also look at the sources of the information. Those sources have motives, and understanding that motive can help decipher the reason for any slant in the information. Equipped with information, the patient can then have an open dialogue with the surgeon or professional whom they're seeking treatment from. Good sources of information include the American Society of Plastic Surgeons (ASPS) and the American Society for Aesthetic Plastic Surgery (ASAPS). There's also my new website, Loopit, for validated patient reviews.

> I do recommend that people considering plastic surgery collect as much data as they can but also look at the sources of the information.

Even more than technological advances, education is paramount to the future of plastic surgery to improve outcomes and for patients to be happier. In the future, we may see any number of technological advances help improve a procedure or the intended outcome, but none of that is as important as making the patient happy, and that will only come with more education.

Developments in Technology and Techniques (The Basic Sciences)

Many of the advancements in education and technology may be the results of plastic surgery being a creative field. The better the technology, the equipment, and the products, the more creative and more advanced the procedures become.

Here are some that we're seeing in the industry today.

- **Skin care.** Improving the longevity of skin is currently at the forefront of today's cosmetic plastic surgery. We're starting to address this earlier, in younger people, and being more aggressive about preventive treatments. It's really never too early to look at ways to protect the skin from the sun and the environment. It's never too early to teach young children to reapply sunblock throughout the day. We're seeing young adults in their twenties getting skin-care treatments to maintain their youthful skin, which is a big deviation from twenty or thirty years ago, when people used to lie in the sun tanning with mirrors directed at their faces and with baby oil on their skin. Healthy skin is becoming a prized value, and it's seen as something beautiful, not something that must always be tan.

- **Loose skin.** The tightening of skin and tissue continues to be a major challenge, so starting early is the best defense for later in life. Unfortunately, there are still no solutions for loose skin; there are no exercises that can tighten skin after a major weight loss. That's frustrating, of course, for people who lose a lot of weight later in life—they may feel a lot healthier and younger, and they certainly look thinner, but they often look older in the face because of all the loose skin. For older folks, there are energy-based therapies to continue to improve skin tightening all through the face and the body.

- **Natural appearance.** We're seeing a reversal of some trends in plastic surgery. For instance, for many years, women wanted larger breasts, even sometimes to the point of looking unnaturally large. But these days, we're removing many breast implants because women want to look more natural. That appears to be a trend with other areas of the body as well, and even when someone undergoes a procedure, they often want the end result to look very natural.

- **Minimal downtime.** As we all know, people can be impatient. We've become a world accustomed to instant answers, so people expect the same with plastic surgery. Although the body takes time to heal, patients today are looking for procedures that produce the maximum results with the minimum downtime.

- **Combination therapy.** Instead of looking at one procedure to provide all the answers, people are starting to see how combining therapies can produce a cumulative result.

- **Energy-based technologies.** There are a number of energy-based technologies using radio frequencies or lasers for therapies that work internally on the body as well as externally on the skin.

- **Tissue regeneration, cell transfer, and blood products.** The basic science of cosmetic plastic surgery continues to evolve with tissue regeneration as a key focus. Science is looking at ways to use a person's natural tissue to improve their appearance or restore a more youthful look. We're also continuing to look at ways to better use fat cells, which are rich in substances that are very beneficial to the body and skin. Where we used to perform macrofat transfer, which is moving larger fat particles from one area of the body to another, we're now doing micro- and even nano-fat grafting—transferring very small particles to enhance plumpness in the face or other areas of the body. We're also exploring ways to use a patient's own blood and blood products through therapies such as Platelet Rich Plasma (PRP), which involves drawing blood, processing it, and then reinjecting it as a way of aiding in healing and rejuvenation. PRP is a safe procedure because it uses the patient's own blood.

In some ways, we do know what the immediate future will bring in plastic surgery, and we have to be positioned to adapt to changing times and fads that come and go. Currently, one of the biggest requests we're seeing is what are known as butt transfers or Brazilian butt lifts, which are procedures to make the bottom appear bigger. Ten or fifteen years ago, no one would think making an already big butt even bigger would be a good thing. Now, because of the Kardashians and social media, it's one of the most requested procedures. Although it's currently a trend, the reality is that it's leading to a refining of techniques—we've begun to figure out ways to be more efficient at fat grafting and fat transfer, potentially leading to some unforeseen benefits in the future. We saw that same thing a few years ago with lip injections—although that was a trend, it forced research into making better fillers.

The evolution of plastic surgery reminds me of a quote that has been attributed to the pioneering carmaker Henry Ford: "If I had asked people what they wanted, they would have said faster horses." Technology changes to meet demand, but it takes foresight to really evolve. The future of plastic surgery is not about just continuing along with incremental improvements but also using our experience and training to look beyond. Our industry benefits people with more than just cosmetic desires; it also benefits people with traumatic injuries. We're the ones who see patients every day. If we don't look at ways to evolve and better meet patients' needs, then nobody else is going to.

"YOU GET IN
LIFE WHAT YOU
HAVE THE COURAGE
TO ASK FOR."

—OPRAH WINFREY

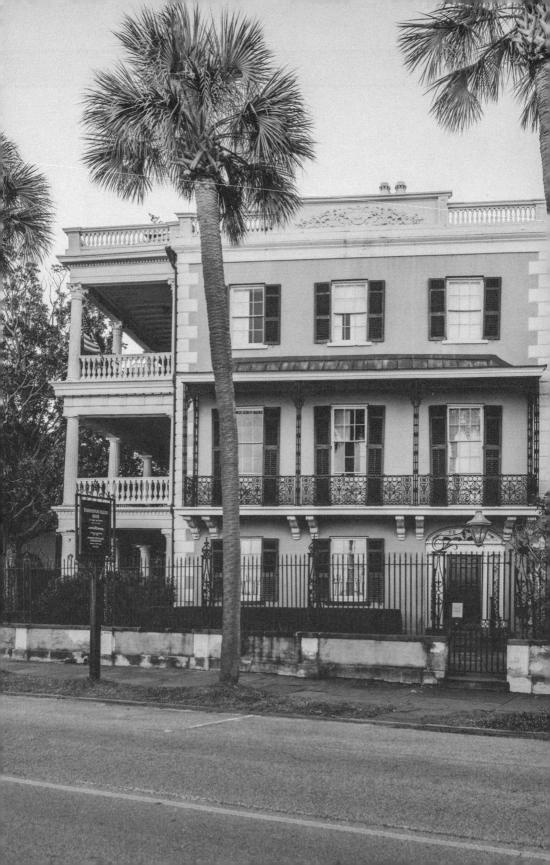

CHAPTER 12

Think, See, or Feel Beauty

Ultimately, what cosmetic plastic patients are looking for, I believe, is "beauty." Whether it is inner or outer beauty, or beauty perceived by someone else, most patients are pursuing some form of self-improvement. When it comes to beauty, most people know it when they encounter it. But ultimately, you can't just think it or see it. In order for it to have a profound and long-lasting impact on your life, it has to be felt.

The definition of beauty changes over time. For instance, what twenty-year-olds think is beautiful will undoubtedly change when they become parents and see their newborns for the first time. And the parents' definition of beauty will change as the children grow and experience life.

As I mentioned in the introduction, my first real, conscious understanding of the concept of beauty came as a result of a TED Talk by product engineer Richard Seymour, who said that consumers buy a product when they connect with it. That connection goes beyond the visual appeal of the product. Consumers buy because of the way a product makes them feel. Out of ten similar products, consumers will choose the one they feel some sort of emotional attachment to.

After hearing that talk, I started thinking about how it applied to plastic surgery. At the time, I was a bit overworked. I thought that if I were to understand my patients better, it would help alleviate some of the stress I was feeling. I asked myself what the people who sought my help were really looking for. The psychology of buying is a subject explored in depth by product and design engineers. However, it is not a subject that doctors tend to focus on. While I was in business school, my area of interest was marketing. I am interested in the emotions concerning choosing a specific product or service. Therefore, I have a better understanding than most other physicians of the concept of buying based on attraction.

When I delved further into the psychology of buying, it dawned on me that there were secondary motivations for having plastic surgery done, and those motivations are very important to each individual. Plastic surgery patients are trying to find beauty in themselves, or they are trying to outwardly improve themselves for someone else, or they are trying to be somebody they never were.

For instance, the woman who always wanted to have a fuller figure and get attention at the beach may have finally reached the age where she has the means to have the body of her dreams. While plastic surgery can give her that body, if she does not adopt a more positive perception of herself, she may discover after the procedure that having more curves is not the answer. Although her body now looks great, she may realize that she still feels unappreciated in spite of getting more attention. The insecurity or unhappiness she has always felt will likely still be present; plastic surgery will not erase those negative feelings. Ironically, as she ages, she may begin to wish she had the more streamlined breasts she had when she was young, before she got implants, and may opt to have the implants removed. The implants she "needed" to be happy she now has to have removed to be happy.

Purchases are driven by emotion. That is human nature, and it is also Apple's secret sauce. Steve Jobs designed Apple products to be about the experience, not just the product's performance or quality. Apple products do not necessarily perform better than other products. In fact, some people might argue that Samsung devices have more features and functions and are more technologically advanced. But the whole experience of having the latest iPhone and being part of the product's cutting-edge branding image strikes an emotional chord in people, which makes them want to purchase the latest similar product, regardless of whether it actually performs better.

The same goes for plastic surgery. On some level, plastic surgery is about trying to deliver an emotion; it is selling hope. It is selling people an answer to their desire to feel good about themselves, to be confident, and to have other people see them as beautiful, in terms of their physical appearances as well as their personalities. It is about selling people the ability to like themselves more. Ideally rather than just an emotional problem, the patient has a problem with a physical feature that leads to unrest or discontent. Cosmetic plastic surgery attempts to address this problem and free the patient from that struggle, ultimately replacing self-doubt with confidence and inner happiness.

So while plastic surgery is commonly thought of as a procedure to address a physical feature of the body, it is just as much about addressing something less tangible: that inner feeling of beauty. It can help people achieve a level of beauty they could not create on their own while alleviating the feeling of insecurity or self-doubt that nags at them.

Once I recognized that plastic surgery is about inner beauty, I began to understand that inner beauty needs to begin early in life.

That led me to start a nonprofit known as Pedals 4 Peanuts. Peanut is my youngest daughter's nickname because she is a very petite child. The idea for Pedals 4 Peanuts began late one December when I was in a big-box store with my oldest daughter, picking up a few last-minute gifts. Among those gifts was a bicycle for Sophia, my youngest daughter, the Peanut. Seeing her excitement on Christmas morning when she unwrapped the bicycle made me realize the impact such a simple gift could have on a child. As her first, new "big girl" bike—it had no training wheels and was not a hand-me-down from one of her older sisters—

> While plastic surgery is commonly thought of as a procedure to address a physical feature of the body, it is just as much about addressing something less tangible: that inner feeling of beauty.

that bike represented more than transportation; it also represented responsibility and independence, a newfound freedom. It was a way for my youngest daughter to begin seeing herself as more of an individual.

Pedals 4 Peanuts provides resources for deserving families to gift their child with their first bicycle and a helmet. The goal of Pedals 4 Peanuts is to help underprivileged kids have a first bike that is truly their own, to give them that same feeling my daughter had that Christmas morning.

Today, the program has expanded to include participation by the local police department in Charleston as a way of building a connection with young kids. The hope is that these kids will remember their first experience with the police as a good one while giving them a reason to be more physically active. At the time of this writing, the organization has given away more than twenty-five hundred new bikes.

Finally, Pedals 4 Peanuts is a way of bringing together two everyday things—a child and a bike—and watching something beautiful happen as a result.

Again, plastic surgery can help improve a feature and change the way you see yourself when you look in a mirror. That can instill more self-confidence. It is ideal for people who want to improve a feature that has been bothering them. It can take them to the next level when they are already on their way to turning their life around. Having a procedure done can also often be a motivator because once people see their physical improvement, they want to keep going and do more to look and feel better. Cosmetic plastic surgery can jump start their journey to being a happier, healthier person overall.

If you want to have cosmetic plastic surgery so that someone will like you more or feel different about you, all you are changing is what that person will see. It will not make someone fall in love with you, it will not make your marriage better, it will not make you enjoy your work more, and it will not make your life perfect. It does not change how others *feel* when they see you, and it will not make someone *feel* that you are a more beautiful person on the inside—and ultimately, that is what lasts.

As a father, especially with four daughters, I often think about the society we live in and the effect that social media is having on today's kids. Two of my daughters are tremendous golfers, obtaining full golf scholarship offers as ninth graders; the other two are competitive gymnasts. In fact, my middle child, Julianna, moved to Texas as a ten-year-old to train at the World Champions Center owned by Nellie Biles and home of Olympian Simone Biles. Julianna trained with Simone on a regular basis, and having watched them practice when I visit, I can say that Simone is hands down the best athlete I have ever personally witnessed. The news stories about her being body shamed on social media were mind boggling to me. That made me think that maybe our job in plastic surgery is as much about helping people achieve their own inner beauty through surgery as it is about helping people realize their beauty in their own skin. Our role is to help fight the cruel and unjust activities that occur on social media and the internet.

Yes, there are risks associated with plastic surgery. That fact cannot be overstated. Plastic surgery is an art, not an exact science. There are no absolute guarantees. But understanding, before the procedure is performed, how a delay in healing or another challenge may be managed can help patients minimize their anxiety after surgery and achieve their desired outcomes.

Simply put, it is a privilege to be a surgeon and take care of people.

But I have seen a dramatic change in the industry and in my ability to perform my job unimpeded, which has been brought about by external factors such as regulations and social media. It's a situation I've seen have a detrimental effect on many surgeons and other health professionals in terms of everything from disenchantment to divorce to drug abuse to suicide.

> It is a privilege to be a surgeon and take care of people.

In fact, rarely a day goes by that someone doesn't ask me if I would do it all over again. Would I spend fifteen years and over one hundred hours a week in training for a job in an industry that has changed so drastically, training for a job that is sometimes rife with frustration and has an inestimable impact on family and personal life? In spite of what people often think, no one initially gets into medicine solely for the money. While we are fortunate to make a good living, there are many other jobs out there making a lot more money for less time commitment and stress. Medical students train first and foremost because they want to help people. They want to make a difference in someone else's life. That's why they push themselves through medical school and residency and then often through some sort of specialty or fellowship.

Perhaps that's why so many physicians and surgeons burn out. Once all the "pushing through" of medical training is over, it would seem there should be more opportunities to keep the momentum going and get out there and set the world on fire, as there are for most graduates of other disciplines. But—especially if a medical graduate goes into private practice—the pressures and responsibilities accumulate. The stress is greater. The financial debt can pile on even more. In the end, the trade-off for all the investment may be a disappointment for some in the healthcare field. It's certainly an eye opener for other business professionals. I learned that while I was in business school pursuing an MBA degree. The other students were dumbfounded at what it takes to run a private medical practice and how dysfunctional overall the healthcare system is today compared to other industries.

Perhaps an even more difficult question I am asked is whether I would encourage any one of my seven children to follow in my footsteps. That's harder to answer because of my natural protective instinct: I want what's best for my kids. Considering the current state of healthcare, I would be hard pressed to tell any one of them that medicine is a good field to enter, especially with the uncertainty all the changes are bringing.

True, there are very few jobs that bring the kind of satisfaction that surgery does. When a surgery goes well and the patient and their loved ones are extremely happy, it's very fulfilling for me as well. Unfortunately, when I encounter patients' misaligned expectations—worsened by social media and society's ever-growing feeling of entitlement—it sometimes seems that the ratio of positive to negative experiences is going in the wrong direction. It is hard today to watch television or go on a social media platform without being inundated with negativity, ranging from political garbage to attention-seeking celebrities. In this day and age, perhaps focusing on ourselves and our own happiness is a way to combat the external forces we have no control over. Once you find your own inner beauty, confidence and happiness will follow.

There is an obvious shift in the world of healthcare, where future generations of doctors and surgeons are going to find it more challenging to deliver care. This is an issue that concerns me because the number of physicians and surgeons burning out or changing careers is already significant. Improving the ability of surgeons and other healthcare professionals to do their jobs will require societal change if the quality of care is to improve rather than decline. After all, we are all getting older by the minute, and we will all need healthcare at some point in the future.

Still, I am excited for the future of plastic surgery. I'm excited that doctors and other healthcare professionals still get into this industry because they want to help others. And I am excited about the possibilities that exist in the field of medicine overall. Ongoing advances in technology are helping to reduce recovery time and the number of setbacks, and improve overall outcomes. By building a relationship with your surgeon and gaining a thorough understanding of the procedure you are undergoing along with its possible challenges, I believe cosmetic plastic surgery can have a significant, positive effect on your life. It can help you find your true beauty, and ultimately help you *become a better you.*

"YOU CAN'T GO BACK
AND CHANGE THE
BEGINNING, BUT YOU
CAN START WHERE
YOU ARE AND CHANGE
THE ENDING."

—C.S. LEWIS

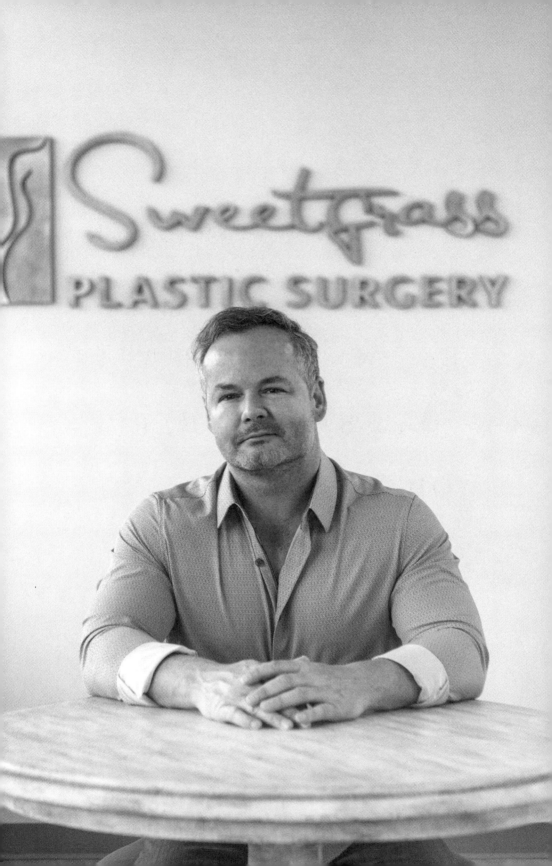

CONCLUSION

A few weeks back, I visited with Olivia, whom I would rate as one of the cutest twelve-year-old girls I've ever seen. Her mother brought her in to see me because she was being teased at school about her ears. Granted, they were a little prominent, but nothing that needed a real fix in a still-growing girl. In truth, they were a feature that may have generated a few comments in her young life, but at some point, one of those comments began to make her self-conscious.

In that consult, I told Olivia that we could do a little something to improve the look of her ears, but ultimately, they were not the problem. The real problem, I explained, was the insecurity of the critics. I hoped that hearing that from a plastic surgeon might help her take my insights a little more to heart. "You're not going to change someone else's view of you by changing something about you based on their criticism," I explained. "You're trying to appease the minority by making a few really deranged people happy." Olivia and her mother laughed and agreed to take a "wait-and-see" attitude.

Now that you've read this book, my hope is that, like Olivia and her mother, you have a better understanding of cosmetic plastic surgery.

Here are a few takeaways I hope you remember for the long term:

- Cosmetic plastic surgery won't change someone else's view of you, and having a procedure to try to make someone see or treat you differently is not the answer. If a school bully is making fun of another child's ears, it's not the ears that need to be changed—it's the bully's outlook. No amount of plastic surgery will change that bully's point of view, which is based on their own insecurities. Some people always find fault in others; that's their objective.

- Cosmetic plastic surgery on its own does not fix feelings of insecurity. When a patient has a self-doubt as a result of a physical imperfection they see in themselves, surgery may change the way they look, and that may give them a new level of self-confidence. But those negative feelings of insecurity or unhappiness may still be present; plastic surgery alone will not erase those.

- Remember: You are your own worst critic. Something you may see as a flaw may be barely visible to or completely overlooked by someone else.

- Patient satisfaction is greatly impacted by the goals for having the surgery—cosmetic plastic surgery will help deliver physical results, but it is the combination of the physical change through the surgery and the patient's newfound self-confidence that ultimately makes a patient feel beautiful.

- Patient perception is key. The best outcomes are those that combine reasonable expectations with personalized procedures that can deliver on those expectations. If you are unsure of the process, start with smaller, less complex procedures, and see the results prior to undergoing further procedures.

- Cosmetic plastic surgery is achievable. So many patients put off having something done because they think that it's unaffordable, complex, and not a solution for something that has bothered them for some time. But there are many, many options today to help turn back the clock or correct any number of issues that people have.

Undergoing cosmetic plastic surgery should not be a necessity for happiness. It is not about trying to mold yourself into something that pleases others or fits what you perceive others to be thinking. It is about what really matters to you. Cosmetic plastic surgery is a great way to change something about yourself that has always been bothersome. No matter what society may say, it's OK to have cosmetic plastic surgery to improve what you see in the mirror.

There are many wonderful options today to make subtle or more dramatic changes, and the right procedures combined with a great outcome and a great outlook help many people improve their self-confidence. And it's that newfound self-confidence that helps project inner happiness to others. That change is what ultimately makes a patient feel beautiful. Because true beauty is not what anyone thinks or sees. It is how *you feel* on the inside.

Remember: It is OK to do something for you. To make a change. It is your life, your body, and you only have one go-round. Make it count.

I wish you the very best in your journey.

Respectfully,

Dennis K. Schimpf, MD, MBA, FACS

Charleston, South Carolina

www.drdennisschimpf.com

www.sweetgrassplasticsurgery.com